DOCUMENTA OPHTHALMOLOGICA

PROCEEDINGS SERIES

Editor

HAROLD E. HENKES

VOL. I

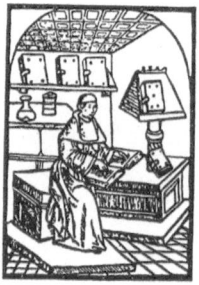

DR. W. JUNK B.V. PUBLISHERS, 1973

THE HAGUE   THE NETHERLANDS

SYMPOSIUM ON LIGHT-COAGULATION

Argon Laser and Xenon Arc

University of Ghent
Department of Ophthalmology
Director: PROF. DR. JULES FRANÇOIS

15–16 June, 1972

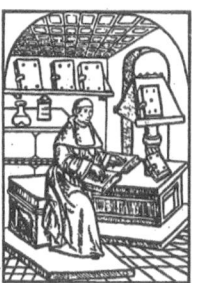

DR. W. JUNK B.V. PUBLISHERS, 1973
THE HAGUE   THE NETHERLANDS

ISBN-13: 978-90-6193-141-6   e-ISBN-13: 978-94-010-2695-6
DOI: 10.1007/ 978-94-010-2695-6

LIST OF REGISTRANTS

ALFIERI, PROF. DR. G., Clinica Oculista. Università, Via P. Giuria 20, Torino, Italy.

AMALRIC, DR. P., Rue St. Clair 6, Albi 81, Tarn, France.

BAY, DR. M., Dept. of Ophthalmology, County Hospital, University of Copenhagen, 2900 Copenhagen, Denmark.

BEC, PROF. DR., 34 Rue Remisat, 31 Toulouse, France.

BEST, DR., Universitäts-Augenklinik, Tübingen, B.R.D.

BINKHORST, DR. P. G., Koninklijk Nederlands Gasthuis voor Ooglijders, F.C. Dondersstraat 65, Utrecht, The Netherlands.

BLACH, DR. R. K., 12 Tylney Avenue, Farguhar Road, London SE 19, England.

BOWBYES, DR. J. A., Moorfields Eye Hospital, City Road, London EC1V 2PD, England.

BRAMBRING, DR. D. F., Löhrstrasse 139, 54 Koblenz, B.R.D.

BREGEAT, PROF. P., 9 rue Théodule-Ribot, Paris XVIIe, France.

BRENIG, DR. H., Alhausstrasse 6, 56 Wuppertal 2, B.R.D.

BRIHAY-VAN GEERTRUYDEN, PROF., St. Pieters Ziekenhuis, Hoogstraat 332, 1000 Brussels, Belgium.

CANENS, DR. A., Utrecht, The Netherlands.

CHABAT-RIVIÈRE, DR., 26 Boulevard Bonne-Nouvelle, Paris Xe, France.

CHAMRAD, DR., Städt. Krankenanstalten, Augenklinik, Heusnerstrasse 40, 56 Wuppertal-Barmen, B.R.D.

CHATELLIER, DR., Centre National d'Ophtalmologie des Quinze-Vingts, 28 Rue de Charenton, Paris XIIe, France.

CHAWLA, DR. H. B., The Royal Infirmary, Princess Alexandra Eye Pavilion, Chalmers-Street, Edinburgh EH3 9HA, Scotland.

CHENG, DR. H., Moorfields Eye Hospital, City Road, London EC1V 2PD, England.

CITRONI, DR. M., Ospedale Civile, Reparto Oculista, Via Taverna 9, Piacenza, Italy.

CLEMETT, DR. R. S., Wellington Avenue 7, Worcester Park, Surrey, England.

CONSTANTINIDES, DR. G., Hôpital Régional, Service d'Ophtalmologie, Cité Hospitalière, 59 Lille, France.

CREMERS, DR., Schoolstraat 6, Utrecht, The Netherlands.

DEBEIR, DR. O., Albertlaan 74, 8300 Knokke, Belgium.

DELLA SIENA, PROF. R. S.

DEMOLDER, DR. E., Tervuerenlaan 194B, 1150 Brussels, Belgium.

DE PALMA, DR. P., Università di Ferrara, Clinica Oculista, Ferrara, Italy.

DERESKEWITZ, DR. J., Augenklinik, Zentralkrankenhaus, St. Jürgen-Strasse, 28 Bremen, B.R.D.

DE ROUCK, DR. A., Antwerpse Steenweg 63, 9110 St. Amandsberg, Belgium.

D'HAENENS, DR. J., E. Beernaertstraat 34, 8400 Oostende, Belgium.

DOLCET BUXERES, DR. LUIS, Muntaner 350, Barcelona, Spain.

EVENS, DR. L., Lakense laan 36, 1090 Brussels, Belgium.

FALCINELLI, PROF. DR. B., Via Francesco Dall'Ongaro 53, Rome, Italy.

FEILER-OFRY, DR. V., Dept. of Ophthalmology, The Chaim Sheba Medical Center, Tel-Hashomer, Israel.

FISON, DR. L., 104 Harley Street, London W1N 1AF, England.

GALLENGA, DR. P. E., Università di Ferrara, Clinica Oculista, Ferrara, Italy.

GARCIA ALIX, DR. CARLOS, General Moscardo 20, Madrid, Spain.

GÄRTNER, PROF. DR. J., Universitäts-Augenklinik Mainz, Langenbeckstrasse 1, 6500 Mainz, B.R.D.

GOES, DR. F., De Roest d'Alkemadelaan 10/H, 2600 Perchem Antwerpen, Belgium.

GUILLAUMAT, PROF. DR. L., Centre National d'Ophtalmologie des Quinze-Vingts, 28 Rue de Charenton, Paris XIIe, France.

HAMILTON, DR. A. M., 22 Moss Close, Pinner Middx, England.

HEIMANN, DR. K., Universitäts-Augenklinik, Lindenburg, 5 Köln-Lindenthal, B.R.D.

HERRERO, DR. and MRS. VIDAL A., Avda. de Cadiz 4, Sevilla, Spain.

HEWSON, DR. G. E., The Crescent, Galway, England.

HOEVENER, DR. G., Klinikum Steglitt, Augenklinik, Hindenbürgdamm 30, 1 Berlin 45, B.R.D.

HOLLWICH, PROF. DR., Universitäts-Augenklinik, 15 Westring, Münster/Westfalen 44, B.R.D.

HOPPENBROUWERS, DR. R., Ooglijdersgasthuis, F.C. Dondersstraat 65, Utrecht, The Netherlands.

HÜBNER, DR. H., Kleiner Eiderkamp 18, 23 Kiel-Schulensee, B.R.D.

IRISARRI, DR. J. P., Clinica Oftalmologica, Avda Generalisimo 606 bajos, Barcelona 15, Spain.

JENS, DR. E., Øjenafdelingen, Rigshospitalet, Blegdamsvej 9, Copenhagen Ø 2100, Denmark.

KAMMANN, DR. J., Baeumerstrasse 26, 46 Dortmund, B.R.D.

KENG SIONG ONG, DR., Augenklinik, Zentralkrankenhaus, St. Jürgen-Strasse 28 Bremen, B.R.D.

KERN, DR. RUDOLF, Augenklinik Kantonalspital, 6000 Lucerne, Switzerland.

KLÖTI, PROF. DR. R., Rosenbühlstrasse 31, Zurich 8044, Switzerland.

KOHNER DR. E., Moorfields Eye Hospital, City Road, London EC1V 2PD, England.

KREISSIG, DR. I., Universitäts-Augenklinik, Venusberg, 53 Bonn 1, B.R.D.

LEUENBERGER, DR. A., Universitäts-Augenklinik, Mittlere Strasse 91, 4000 Basel, Switzerland.

LEVY, DR. D., 1 Rue Bonaparte, Paris VIIe, France.

LIEB, PROF. DR. W., Städt. Krankenhaus Höchst, 6230 Frankfurt a. Main 80. B.R.D.

MARSAULT, DR. M., 112 Rue du Bac, Paris VIIe, France.

MASSIN, DR. M., 5 Villa Jocelyn (Square Lamertine), Paris XVIe, France.

NAUTNER, DR. W., Medizinische Akademie, Ratzeburger Allee 160, 24 Lübeck, B.R.D.

MENEZO, DR. JOSE LUIS, Jorge Juan 6, 8°, Valencia, Spain.

MERIN, DR. S., Dept. of Ophthalmology, Hadassah Medical Organization, Mayer de Rothschild Hadassan, University Hospital, Jerusalem, Israel.

MERTENS, DR. D. A. E., Dept. of Ophthalmology, Rotterdam Medical Faculty, Schiedamse Vest 180, Rotterdam 3001, The Netherlands.

MILANO, DR. M. L., Ospedali Riuniti di Napoli, Divisione Oculista, Via Cardarelli 9, Napoli, Italy.

MILDNER, DR. I., Spandauer Damm 130, 1 Berlin 19, B.R.D.

MILLER, DR. H., 19 Boulevard Beauséjour, Paris XVIe, France.

OLIVELLA, DR. A., Clinica Oftalmologia, Avda Generalisimo 606 bajos, Barcelona 15, Spain.

ORTBAUER, DR. R., Im Sommerwind 13a, 7 Stuttgart-Vaihingen, B.R.D.

PANNARALE, DR. M. R., Via dei Monti Parioli 28, Rome, Italy.

PAPADOPOULOS, DR. P., 1 Neofronos St., Athens T 508, Greece.

PARREN, DR. H. G., Herenlaan 7, Zeist, The Netherlands.

PAUL, DR., Städt. Krankenhaus Höchst, 6230 Frankfurt a. Main 80, B.R.D.

PERRIAM, DR. D. J., 53 Rosebery Gardens, London N8 8SH, England.

QUIST, DR.

RABAEY, PROF. DR. M., Watervallestraat 71, 9150 Grembergen, Belgium.

RENARDEL DE LAVALETTE, DR. J. G. C., Dept. of Ophthalmology, Rotterdam Medical Faculty, Schiedamse Vest 180, Rotterdam 3001, The Netherlands.

RICHARD, DR. Y., 14 Rue Taine, Paris XIIe, France.

RINALDI, DR. G., Via Sergio Laghi 2, 1° p., Trieste, Italy.

ROSENBERG, DR. TH., Dept. of Ophthalmology, County Hospital Gentofte, University of Copenhagen, DK 2900 Hellerup, Denmark.

ROUCHY, DR. J. P., Dép. d'Ophtalmologie, Hôpital de la Croix Seint-Simon, 11 Avenue Elisée Reclus, Paris VIIe, France.

SAKAVE, PROF. DR. E., Kyoto University Faculty of Medecine, Dept. of Ophthalmology, Kyoto, Japan.

SAND, DR. A. BRATBERG, Dept. of Ophthalmology, Ulleval Sykehus, Oslo, Norway.

SCHEFFER, DR. C. H., 1e Brandenburgerweg 14, De Bilt, The Netherlands.

SCHILDBERG, DR. P., Städt. Krankenanstalten, Augenklinik, Hufelandstrasse 55, 4300 Essen-Holsterhausen, B.R.D.

SCHMALFUSS, DR. C., Städt. Krankenanstalten, Augenklinik, Hufelandstrasse 55, 4300 Essen-Holsterhausen, B.R.D.

SCHWIND, DR. H. B., Städt. Krankenhaus Höchst, 6230 Frankfurt a. Main 80, B.R.D.

SEEDORFF, DR. H. H., Rigshospitalet, Afdelingen for Øjensygdomme, Tagensvej 18, 2200 Copenhagen N, Denmark.

STRAMPELLI, PROF. B., Corso d'Italia, Rome, Italy.

THOMANN, PROF. DR. H., Augenklinik, St. Josefs-Hospital, Friedenstrasse 24, 58 Hagen, B.R.D.

TRANOS, DR. L., 5 Rue Herodou Attikou, Athens, Greece.

TREISTER, DR. G., Dept. of Ophthalmology, The Chaim Sheba Medical Center, Tel-Hashomer, Israel.

TSOLAKIS G. PANAYOTIS, DR., Solones 44, T 135, Athens, Greece.

ULLERICH, PROF. DR. K., Augenklinik, Städt. Krankenanstalten, 40 Beurhausstrasse, 46 Dortmund, B.R.D.

URRETS-ZAVALLA, PROF. A., Casilla de Correo 301, Cordoba, Argentine.

VAN DEN HEUVEL, PROF. J. E. A., Ophthalmological Clinic, Geert Groteplein Zuid 22, Nijmegen, The Netherlands.

VAN OYE, DR. R., Kortrijkse Steenweg 251, 9830 St. Martens-Latem, Belgium.

VERRIEST, DR. G., Coupure 79, 9000 Ghent, Belgium.

VERSTREPEN, DR. S., Dijkstraat 17, 9330 Dendermonde, Belgium.

VERZELLA, DR. F., Corso Porta Mare 11, Ferrara, Italy.

VON WINNING, DR. C. H. O. M., Wassenaarse weg 29, The Hague, The Netherlands.

ZARETSKI, DR. M., 78 Rue Brillat Savarin, Paris XIIIe, France.

ZARRABI, DR., Hôpital des Quinze-Vingts, 13 Rue Moreau, 75 Paris XIIe, France.

CONTENTS

INTRODUCTION

The purpose of this symposium on light-coagulation is not to show the superiority of the argon-laser-coagulation or, on the contrary, of the classical photocoagulation, but rather to see, if possible, which are the respective indications and contraindications for xenon-arc-coagulation as well as for argon-laser-coagulation.

So, for instance, the argon-laser-coagulator is perhaps more appropriate to treat the lesions at and around the macula and the optic disc, but for the peripheral lesions of the retina the xenon-arc photocoagulator is surely as effective. For the conservative treatment of intraocular tumours, the xenon-arc-coagulator is beyond doubt more efficacious than the argon-laser-coagulator.

We were very happy to have at this symposium Professor MEYER-SCHWICKERATH, the creator and the pioneer of light-coagulation, his coworker, Professor WESSING, and Doctor HUNTER LITTLE, one of the pioneers of the laser-therapy. We thank them very warmly for having brought to us the results of their prominent clinical experiments.

After general considerations on laser-photocoagulation, we will have a discussion on macular alterations and their treatment as well as on peripheral retinal vascular or non vascular diseases. The most important part concerns the treatment of diabetic retinopathy. Finally the prevention of complications in argon laser retinal photocoagulation will be reviewed.

In conclusion, this symposium gives us a synthesis of what we know at the present time about light coagulation with the help of the xenon arc as well as of the argon laser. I hope that these information will be of great educational value for ophthalmologists.

Professor JULES FRANÇOIS

LIGHT, LASERS AND OCULAR PHOTOCOAGULATION

J. FRANÇOIS & E. CAMBIE

(Ghent)

To understand the properties of the lasers, we will first see how lasers operate and how they differ from all the previous sources of light.

Before the lasers, all light was essentially generated by hot bodies of one or another kind, whether it was the sun or the filament of an incandescent lamp.

Regular light sources emit many wavelengths, what means continuous distribution of wavelengths. If a single pure colour is needed, it can be obtained only by filtering out all the other wavelengths, and usually there is not much power remaining. This is the reason why a xenon arc can never be modified to emit monochromatic light, which would be powerfull enough to be used for photocoagulation. A laser, on the other hand, emits all its power at a single wavelength or frequency.

Ordinary light sources are really not very powerfull although some of them appear very bright to our sensitive eyes. The unfocused sunlight on the earth has a power density of 100 milliwatt/mm^2 and when focused, a maximal power density of 1,7 W/mm^2.

It is well known that when two waves, having the same wavelength, arrive simultaneously at the same place, they may add or substract depending on whether they are in or out of phase.

Light is called coherent if its waves are of the same length, and are going in the same direction. Coherent means ordered. When the waves are not parallel and the wavelengths different, the light is incoherent.

Lasers can generate light that is highly coherent. They do so, because the numerous individual atoms in their active media are forced to emit in phase instead of to emit randomly. The word 'Laser' is an acronym of 'Light Amplification by Stimulated Emission of Radiation'.

From the nature itself of laser light, we can deduce its properties, which are primarily monochromaticity and a high degree of focusability (Fig. 1). Concerning the interactions with biological material, the absorption characteristics of the tissues are relatively broad and there is no need for very narrow spectral width.

From the Ophthalmological Clinic of the University of Ghent. Director: Prof. J. FRANÇOIS.

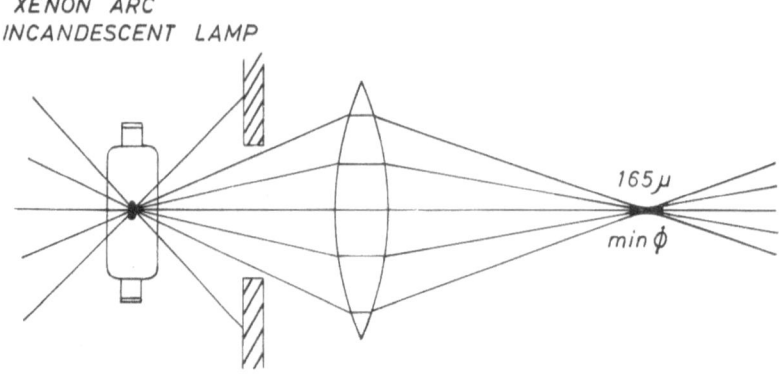

XENON ARC
INCANDESCENT LAMP

165μ

min φ

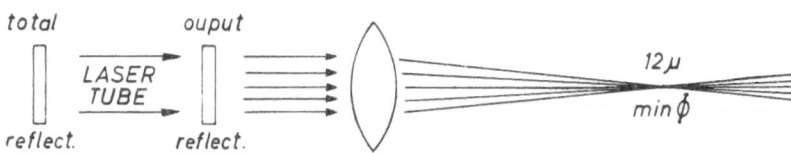

total   ouput

LASER
TUBE

12μ

min φ

reflect.   reflect.

Fig. 1. The focusing is better with a laser light than with a xenon arc or incandescent lamp. The smallest theoretical spotsize with the xenon arc will be 165 μ, and with the commercially available argon laser 12 μ.

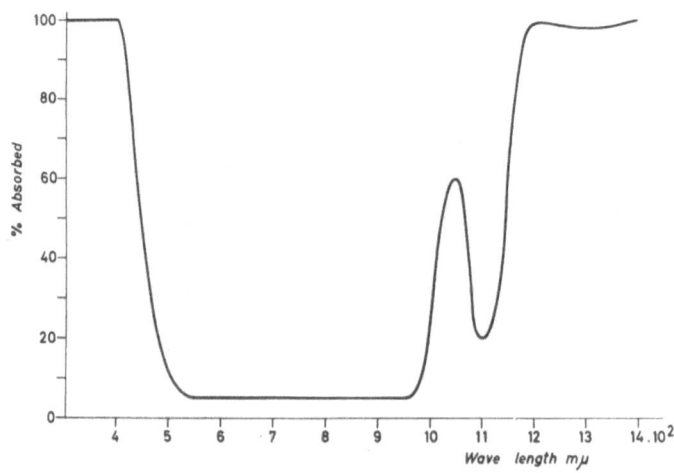

Fig. 2. Ocular transmission curve.

Only light sources which emit wavelengths nearly not absorbed by the ocular media but highly absorbed by the ocular pigments (melanin and haemoglobin) can be used for photocoagulation.

Only the wavelengths between 4.000 and 14.000 Å are transmitted by the ocular media. The highest transmission rate is between 5.000 and 9.000 Å. The short wavelengths are absorbed by the cornea, the long wavelengths by the water of the media and the lens (Fig. 2).

The melanin granules absorb all the transmitted light but mainly in the range between 4.500 and 8.500 Å. Haemoglobin absorbs all the transmitted wavelengths till 6.000 Å.

Superimposing the ocular transmission curve on this of the melanin, responsible for the major part of the absorption in the pigment epithelium and the choroid, and on this of haemoglobin, we may conclude that only light sources with a wavelength between 4.500 and 6.000 Å are the most appropriate for ocular photocoagulation (Fig. 3). The fall-off on the short wavelength end is due to the decrease in transmission characteristics of the eye, the fall-off on the long wavelength end is due to the abrupt decrease of haemoglobin absorption. This means that a blue, green or yellow laser can selectively coagulate the melanin and the haemoglobin (Fig. 4), while the red lasers and the xenon arc with emission of long wavelength light in the red spectrum can only selectively coagulate the melanin. Coagulation of the pigment epithelium with secondary coagulation of the blood vessels by heat irradiation is also possible (Fig. 5).

As we know the energy of a photon varies with the inverse proportion of the wavelength. Therefore it is not surprising that interactions with biological

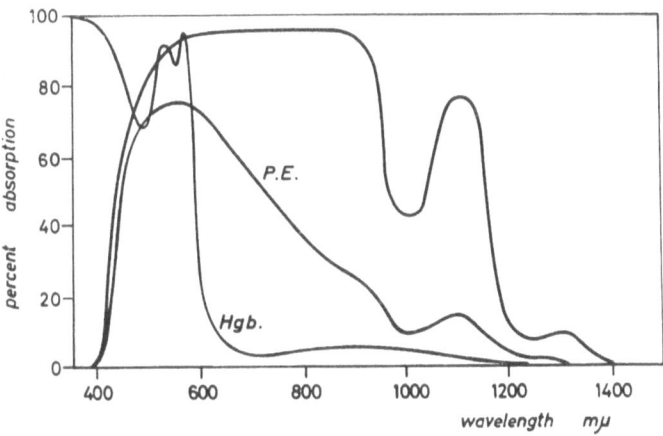

Fig. 3. The ocular transmission curve superimposed on the absorption curve for haemoglobin and melanin.

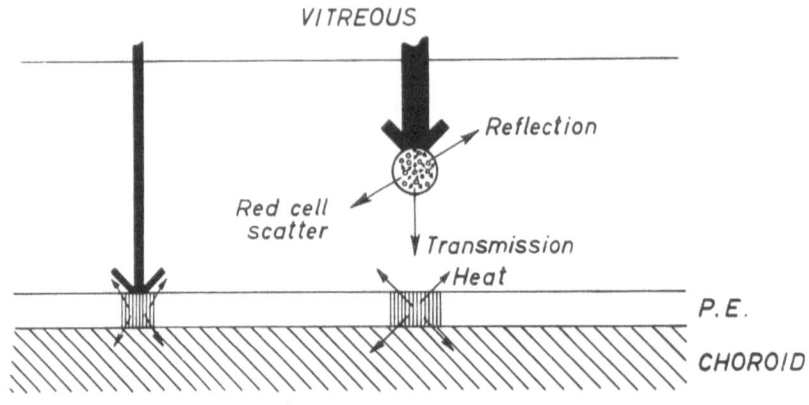

Fig. 4. Direct photocoagulation with the argon laser of the pigment epithelium and the bloodvessels.

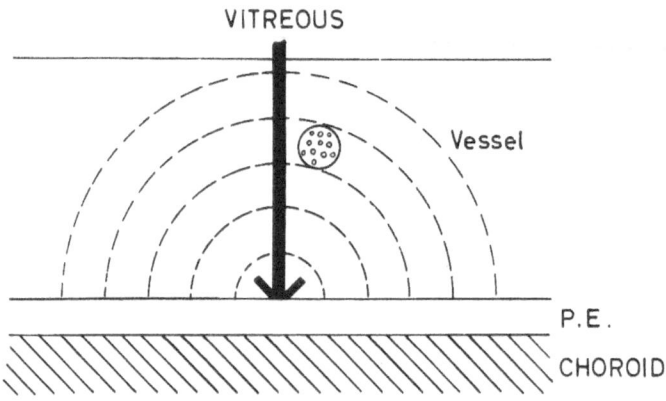

Fig. 5. Direct photocoagulation with the ruby laser or the xenon arc of the pigment epithelium and secondary (indirect) coagulation of the bloodvessels by heat irradiation from the pigment epithelium.

material are quite different depending on the wavelength. In the low spectral range there is, besides the photothermal effect, a more pronounced photochemical effect than in the long spectral range. This means that the blue green laser, when it is focused in the retina or the vitreous, has more tendency to produce biochemical alterations than the red laser light.

Because of the low absorption in the red part of the spectrum, the ruby laser will be absorbed less than the blue green laser (Table I).

Table I. *Absorption of light by ocular media.*

Source	Absorption
Ruby	6%
Neodymium Q switched	6%
Krypton	6–13%
Argon	12%
Xenon arc	24%
Neodymium	35%

PRINCIPLES OF PHOTOCOAGULATION

The smallest obtainable unit of light energy is the photon. The light intensity varies with the photonflux in the beam. When absorbed by pigments these photons give thermal interactions. This thermal damage, caused by the fact that the photons are absorbed and converted into heat, is at the basis of the coagulation of biological tissues (photocoagulation).

TYPES OF LASERS

There are four types of lasers, which could be used for photocoagulation (Table II):
1. Continuous wave gas lasers.
2. Pulsed or Q-switched solid state lasers.
3. Pulsed gas lasers or burst lasers.
4. Continuous wave dye lasers.

Table II. *Types of lasers.*

1. *Continuous wave gas lasers*
   a. Argon laser: (6 W laser) 4579 Å and 5145 Å
   b. Helium-neon laser: (50 mW laser) 6328 Å
   c. Krypton laser: (500 mW laser) 4785 Å (50 mW)
   5308 Å (50 mW)
   5682 Å (50 mW)
   6471 Å (350 mW)

2. *Pulsed solid state lasers*
   a. Ruby laser: (15 W laser) 6943 Å
   b. Neodymium doped YAG laser: (1000 W laser) 10.600 Å
   c. Neodymium Q-switched laser (10–20 W laser) 5.300 Å

3. *Burst laser*
   Pulsed argon laser (1 W laser) 4579 Å and 5145 Å

4. *Dye lasers or liquid lasers*
   Dye laser with argon laser (6 W) as a pump (maximally 50 mW): 5600 Å till 6500 Å.

I. *Continuous wave gas lasers*

The gas lasers are characterized by a continuous emission of laser light. The exposure time is unlimited and the spotsize can be regulated from less than 1 micron to several mm. Three types are available for photocoagulation.

a. *Argon laser*

The argon laser is a 6 W laser (maximal 3 W on the cornea) with an emission of laser light of six lines between 4579 and 5145 Å. However only the 4880 and 5145 Å lines, which contain more than 80% of the energy output, are powerfull enough to give a good oedematous reaction.

At very low power, mainly the blue component is emitted and at high power, both components are emitted with equal power. The high power on continous wave basis, and the high absorption by melanin and haemoglobin makes it a very useful laser for photocoagulation, where mainly intensities between 50 and 500 mW are used during 0,01 second or more.

b. *Helium-neon laser*

The helium-neon laser is a 50 mW laser (maximal 25 mW on the cornea) with an emission of red light (6328 Å). This laser is not appropriate for photocoagulation because of its low energy output.

c. *Krypton laser*

The krypton laser has an emission spectrum of four different main wavelengths (4785, 5308, 5682 and 6471 Å), which can be separately selected by using a prism wavelength selector. The various intensities are too low to be used for a normal photocoagulation. A maximum power of 350 mW is available in the red and one of 50 mW in the yellow, the green and the blue line. But a krypton laser with sufficient power for the full spectrum of photocoagulation treatments would be too expensive.

In conclusion, among the gas lasers only the argon laser is clinically useful at the present time.

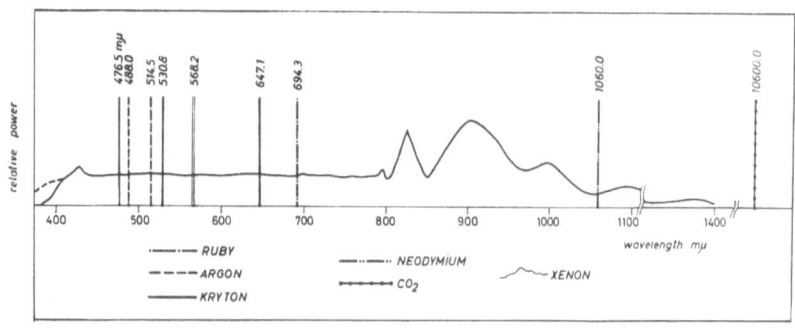

Fig. 6. Emission spectra of the xenon arc and the different lasers.

2. Pulsed solid state lasers

Solid state lasers are characterized by a pulsed emission of laser light. The pulse length cannot be varied and between each pulse one has to wait 5 till 10 seconds in order to charge the capacitors and to cool the system. This makes already the gas lasers superior because of their continuous wave nature, avoiding bursting lesions of the retina.

There are two types of solid state lasers available.

a. Ruby laser

The ruby laser is a 15 watt laser with a constant exposure time of about 0.5 msec, an emission wavelength of 6.943 Å and a spotsize of 100 to 500 μ varying from one instrument to another.

b. Neodymium laser

The neodymium laser is a 1 kw laser with a constant exposure time of about 1 msec and an emission wavelength of 10.600 Å. This can be halved to 5.300 Å by a doubling crystal, the peak power being only 10 to 20 W. The disadvantages of this Q-switched laser is that the doubling crystal is subject to thermal damage, that the neodymium pump lamps have only a lifetime of about 100 hours, that there is an energy loss from 1000 W to 10–20 W and that the price is 50% higher than for other lasers (Fig. 7). For these practical reasons at the present time the neodymium laser will not become a useful photocoagulator.

3. Burst lasers

The burst lasers are 1 W gas lasers (maximal 0,5 W at the cornea), using for example argon and operating in a pulsed mode, whereby the repetition rate may be increased for short bursts to produce a sufficient average power for coagulation (Fig. 8).

In this way they reduce the power consumption and only air cooling is necessary. The great disadvantage is the non continuous emission (what makes of a gas laser a solid state laser with pulsed emission). Moreover, this laser has only one sixth of the power capacity of the commercial available continuous wave argon laser.

The disadvantage of burst lasers, as well as of pulsed lasers, is the danger of retinal micro-explosions due to the excessive peak power by small exposure times and this is an important disability when peroperative haemorrhages occur.

4. Dye lasers or liquid lasers

These are tuneble lasers, which use a 6 W argon laser as a pump and can produce colours from yellow through red. The selection of the colour will be made by turning prisms (Fig. 9). The big disadvantage is the very low power output (only 10 to 50 mW).

7

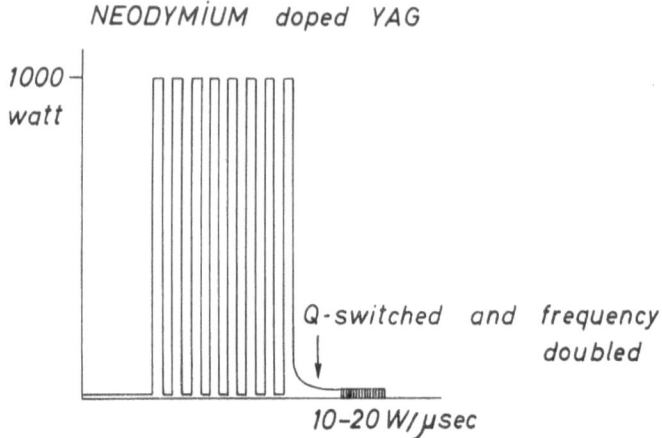

Fig. 7. Scheme to illustrate the loss of power due to Q switching and frequency doubling of the neodymium doped YAG laser.

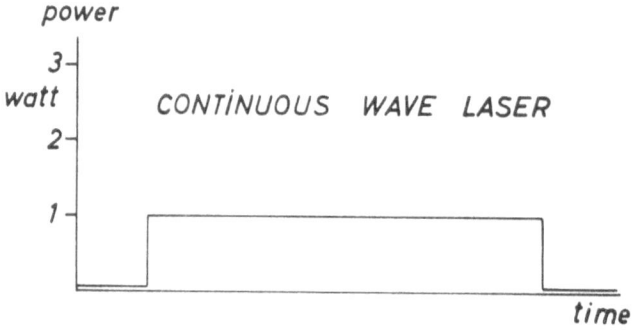

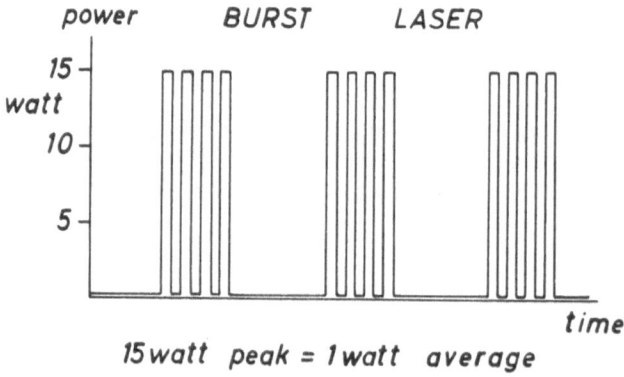

Fig. 8. Difference between the argon continuous laser and the argon burst laser.

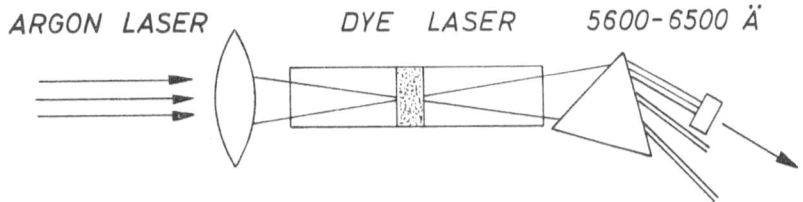

Fig. 9. The dye laser, stimulated by an argon gas laser, emits different wavelengths, which can be selected by rotating a prism behind the output reflector.

In conclusion, only two lasers are really useful for ocular photocoagulation: the ruby laser, which is a pulsed solid state laser, and the argon laser, which is a continuous gas laser. The great advantages of the argon laser over the ruby laser are:

1. Uniform coagulation spots (no hot spots).
2. Free choice of spot size.
3. Free choice of exposure duration.
4. High absorption in both haemoglobin and melanin.
5. Less danger of micro-explosions of the retina.
6. Identical aiming and operating beam.
7. Possibility for fluorescein activation.
8. Excellent visibility of the retina during exposure.
9. Continuous wave nature.

The advantages of laser light over xenon arc light are due to its monochromaticity and spatial coherence, what allows:

1. Optimal focalisation.
2. Exact and small spotsize determination.
3. Acurate power control.
4. Lower absorption by the ocular media.

PRINCIPLES AND INDICATIONS FOR SLIT LAMP ARGON LASER PHOTOCOAGULATION

J. FRANÇOIS & E. CAMBIE

(Ghent)

In principle the indications of argon laser photocoagulation are the same as for xenon arc photocoagulation, with the exception of glaucoma surgery, iridotomy and trabecular meshwork destruction (Table I), and the treatment of intravitreal or prepapillary vascular neoformation as well as of macular lesions close to the fovea (Table III).

We use the slit lamp photocoagulator in all the cases because of the wide field, the high magnification, the stereoscopic view and the comfortable position for the patient as well as for the doctor.

Table I. *Indications for argon laser photocoagulation. Anterior segment.*

Eye lids: xanthelasma, naevi, angiomas, papillomas.
Conjunctiva: naevi, angiomas, papillomas, subconjunctival haemorrhages.
Cornea: ulcers, neovascularisation.
Iris: iris prolaps, iris cysts, corepraxis, iridotomy.
Anterior chamber angle: trabecular meshwork.

I. ANTERIOR SEGMENT OF THE EYE

For photocoagulation of the eyelids the energy requested is much higher (till 3 Watts) than for the other ocular structures. For this reason a local anesthesia is necessary. The lesions disappear after one or more sessions without any scar formation.

For conjunctival, corneal, iris and anterior chamber angle photocoagulation, energies lower than 1 W are requested and only a topical anesthesia is necessary.

For corneal neovascularisation a 50 μ spotsize and energies of 100–300 W are always used with short exposure times to avoid corneal damage. The treatment of corneal ulcers after fluorescein activitation is more a theoretical than a really practical application.

For iris photocoagulation the energy requested depends mainly on the amount of iris pigmentation and the purpose of the treatment.

From the Ophthalmological Clinic of the University of Ghent. Director: Prof. J. FRANÇOIS.

Iris prolaps: 100 or 200 µ spotsize and energies varying from 100–300 mW.

Iris cysts: after surgical or laser (50 µ spot at high energy) puncture of the cyst, a 100 µ spotsize with energies till 1 W is needed for the destruction of the collapsed cyst.

Corepraxis: a 200 or 500 µ spotsize and an energy of 200 till 500 mW are needed, while focusing on the iris base. If small spotsizes and high power are used, lens damage may happen.

Iridotomy: a 50 µ spotsize, high intensities and a very short exposure time (maximally 0,1 sec.) are needed. In the first session only a destruction of the iris stroma with immediate pigment accumulation and gas bubble formation is obtained. Only in the second session the pigmented scar and the iris pigment layer will be perforated. In phakic patients the coagulation has to be done with the Goldmann three mirror contact lens, using the large mirror for the midperiphery to direct the beam more tangentially to the iris basis and to diminish the chance for cataract formation. In aphakic patients a direct photocoagulation throughout the contact lens may be done. In all the cases of iris photocoagulation a severe fibrinous reaction occurs immediately after the treatment, but disappears without any complication after a two days local corticosteroid application.

For trabecular meshwork destruction, we tried, in one or more sessions, to make the way free to Schlemm's canal, but without convincing results. We used a 50 µ spotsize and high intensities till 1 Watt. Angle coagulation, with or without fluorescein activation and with or without jugular vein compression, does not give the expected results at the present time.

2. POSTERIOR SEGMENT OF THE EYE

In all the cases a regular Goldmann contactlens or a three mirror Goldmann lens was used, what offers the advantage to be able to explore and to treat all the areas of the retina.

We are mainly concerned with retinal and choroidal alterations. For the retina the power settings and spotsize determination are dependent on the transparency of the ocular media, the amount of pigmentation, the thickness of the bloodvesselwall and the physiopathology of the lesion.

The amount of pigmentation differs not only from one case to another, but depends also on the localisation in the retina. The melanin granules are denser in the macular and peripapillar zone than in the midperiphery or in the extreme periphery. A continuous adjustment of power settings or exposure times is necessary to avoid complications due to excessive power density. This means that in a non- Caucasian a reaction can be seen with 50 mW, while in a blond Caucasian the same reaction is only seen with 100 or 150 mW. Even in the same eye the intensity may be 100 mW in the macular region to obtain a lesion similar to that obtained in the periphery with 150 mW.

Another important fact is the degree of elevation of the pigment epithelium and the nature of the underlying pathology. Haemorrhagic pigment epithelium detachments need less energy density than serous pigment epithelium detachment, because in the first case the melanin as well as the haemoglobin absorb the argon laser light. If the detachment is too extensive and too elevated it will be unwise to coagulate the lesion and only a barrage around this has to be done.

For bloodvessel coagulation lower energy is needed to coagulate veins than arteries because of the difference in thickness of the bloodvessel wall, but the energy has to be at least two times higher than for pigment lesions. Otherwise only a spasm of the vessels is obtained and not a full obstruction. The obliteration of the vessel can be reinforced by coagulating the underlying pigment-epithelium, which gives an oedematoes reaction around the bloodvessels. Usually we produce first an oedematous reaction around the bloodvessels and then with high energy we focalise on the bloodvessel to create its total obstruction. In this way we avoid choroidal haemorrhages during the eye movement, due to the high power needed for bloodvessel photocoagulation and reaching the pigment epithelium.

Choroidal lesions with rupture of Bruch's membrane, as e.g., in histoplasmosis, angioid streaks or pigment epithelium detachments, need higher power settings because of the fragility of the underlying choroidal capillary vessels. A strong reaction is here needed. Otherwise subepithelial and retinal haemorrhages may occur immediately after the photocoagulation. For this reason it is advised to make first a barrage around the lesion or near the macula to protect the surrounding areas from subepithelial haemorrhages.

The spotsize determination is also very important, because the total amount of energy is exactly the same in a 50 μ than in a 1000 μ spotsize, which means that the energy density on a power setting will be much higher for the 50 μ than for the 1000 μ spot. On the other hand, small spotsizes (50 and 100 μ) are more prone to burst the retina and choroid on high intensities than large spotsizes. It is clear that most complications will appear by high power settings on the 50 or 100 μ spotsize.

Small spotsizes are only used for macular lesions and prepapillar and intravitreal vascular neoformations. Around the macular region, spotsizes of 100 or 200 μ are used, while for the periphery spotsizes of 200 or 500 μ will be used. The advantage of the 50, 100 and 200 μ spotsize is that by regular photocoagulation they do not hurt the patient, while 500 and 1000 μ spotsize do so because of the higher energy output necessary to obtain a similar lesion.

Our immediate complications, choroidal as well as retinal haemorrhages, were due to high power settings with a 50 μ and sometimes 100 μ spotsize. We did not encounter these haemorrhages with the larger spotsizes (200–500–1000 μ).

The advantage of several small coagulation spots instead of a larger one is the possibility of a better thermal cooling. Therefore, we place several 100 or 200 μ spotsizes to obtain the same lesion as with a 1000 μ one. This is probably the reason why vitreous membrane traction is exceptional after argon laser photocoagulation.

Only by low power settings, the spotsize indicated on the marker will be the same in the retina after coagulation. If using higher power, the spotsize will become larger due to the irradiation of heat and this is mainly true for small spotsizes. A 50 μ spot will be a 50 μ spotsize in the retina with 50 mW, but becomes a 100 μ or even 300 μ spotsize by increasing the intensity. There is also a correlation between the amount of oedema and the extension of the lesion into the choroid or the retina.

The intensity requested for obtaining a chorioretinal reaction depends on several factors:

1. The amount of pigmentation of the area to be treated.

2. The transparency of the ocular media.

3. The elevation of the lesion (pigment epithelium detachment) or the surrounding oedema.

4. The localisation of the lesion (intraretinal, intravitreal or choroidal).

5. The thickness of the bloodvessel wall.

To determine the threshold power for photocoagulation, the power has to be increased with small increments in the area to be treated (in contrast to the large increments of the xenon arc). Only after the determination of this power settings, we may increase the intensity to obtain the suitable reaction.

The exposure time, which can be regulated from 0,01 second till continuous, plays also an important role in obtaining the suitable lesion. With low power settings and long exposure time, the same lesion as with higher power settings and short exposure times can be obtained with spotsizes of 200 μ and larger. With small spotsizes (50 and 100 μ), with high power settings and short exposure times, bursts of the retina and the choroid may be obtained with immediate choroidal haemorrhages: with lower intensities and longer exposure times, only an oedematous reaction will occur. Consequently it is not a rule that the same reaction can be obtained when varying the intensity and exposure time. This is also the advantage of continous wave laser or xenon arc over pulsed lasers, which give more frequently retinal and choroidal bursts.

There are three methods of therapy: the direct, the indirect and the combined method (Table II).

The direct method consists in the treatment of the lesion itself, while the indirect method consists in the treatment of areas adjacent to the lesion (barrage) in order to prevent the complications of the direct method. In several diseases a combination of both methods is indicated, as for example in Eales' disease or in diabetes.

The indications of retinal and choroidal argon laser slitlamp photocoagulation are listed in Table III.

The contra-indications for argon laser photocoagulation are the lack of transparency of the ocular media: corneal haziness, pigment deposits on the corneal endothelium interfering with the laser beam, cataract (mainly the nuclear form) and vitreous alterations (fibrous tissue, remnants of haemorrhages). The amount of interference of the ocular media can easily be judged by the diffraction of the laser light on the retinal lesion and by the power setting necessary to obtain a reaction.

Table II. *Indications of the different methods of photocoagulation.*

I. *Direct Method*
1. Serous central retinopathy
2. Pigment epithelium detachment
3. Rupture of the Bruch's membrane
4. Histoplasmosis
5. Diabetes
6. Eales' disease
7. Coats' disease

II. *Indirect Method*
1. Diabetes
2. Eales' disease
3. Peripheral degenerations predisposing to retinal detachment
4. Retinoschisis, retinal cysts
5. Venous branch thrombosis

III. *Combined Method*
1. Diabetes
2. Eales' disease

Table III. *Indications for argon laser slitlamp photocoagulation.*
Posterior segment.

I. *Vascular anomalies*
1. Diabetes
2. Eales' disease
3. Coats' disease
4. Venous branch obstruction with macular oedema
5. Sickle cell retinopathy
6. Retrolental fibroplasia

II. *Peripheral lesions*
1. Retinal holes, tears, cystic degeneration (without detachment)
2. Retinoschisis and retinal cysts

III. *Macular lesions*
1. Central serous retinopathy
2. Pigment epithelium detachment
3. Rupture of Bruch's membrane
4. Choroidal inflammations extending into the retina (histoplasmosis)
5. Secondary macular oedema

A pupil size smaller than 5 mm is a second contra-indication, because of the risk of iris-sphincter coagulation with local cataract formation.

Patients under anticoagulantia and patients with large fluorescein leaking areas into the vitreous may not be treated immediately. Anticoagulantia have to be stopped for at least 3 days before the treatment. When there are large areas of fluorescein diffusion, one has to wait 2 days after the fluorescein angiography; otherwise the fluorescein, diffused in the vitreous, enhances the argon laser light absorption, so that there is a risk of vitreous heating, fibrous tissue formation and vitreous membrane retraction.

ARGON LASER RETINAL PHOTOCOAGULATION: INSTRUMENTATION AND GENERAL TECHNIQUES

HUNTER L. LITTLE, M.D.

(Palo Alto, California)

Currently there are five commercially available argon laser photocoagulators for use in ophthalmology. All are manufactured by the following companies in the United States:

Britt Electronic Products Corp., 2944 Nebraska Ave., Santa Monica, California.

Coherent Radiation, 932 East Meadow Drive, Palo Alto, California 94303.

Lynex Incorporated, 3726 Lonsdale Street, Cincinnati, Ohio 45227.

Medical Instrument Research Associates, Inc., 150 Causeway Street, Boston, Massachusetts 02114.

Optics Technology, Inc., Stanford Industrial Park, Palo Alto, California 94304.

Table I summarizes the data of the five instruments noting the type and power of the laser, the power available to the eye, the delivery system, the spot size range, the exposure time range, and the cooling source.

All of the instruments are available with the slit lamp delivery systems which provide binocular viewing with adequate illumination and magnification. With the three mirror contact lens one can treat lesions from the macula to the ora serrata. The author finds that the direct and monocular indirect delivery systems offer little advantage over the slit lamp delivery systems. When scleral depression is required, the author usually prefers to use transconjunctile cryosurgery viewed with binocular indirect ophthalmoscopy.

The initial instrumentation of the argon laser slit lamp photocoagulator was made possible through a National Institutes of Health research grant (LITTLE, ZWENG & PEABODY, 1970). A team consisting of Dr. H. C. ZWENG, Dr. HUNTER L. LITTLE, and Dr. ROBERT R. PEABODY as ophthalmologists and Dr. ARTHUR VESSILIATES, an electrical engineer, and Mr. NORMAN PEPPERS, and optical engineer, was organized for the project. After three years of research and development of the instrument at Stanford Research Institute, a commercial company Coherent Radiation Laboratories then made the commercial model in production today. None of the above named physicians are in any way affiliated with Coherent Radiation other than as consultants on the photocoagulation project.

A comparative evaluation of the various argon laser photocoagulators is

Palo Alto Medical Clinic, Palo Alto Medical Research Foundation and Stanford University School of Medicine, Palo Alto, California.

Table I.

Argon Laser Photocoagulators	Type Laser	Cooling	Power (milliwatts)	Retinal Spot Size (microns)	Exposure Time (seconds)	Delivery Systems
Britt	pulsed 3000/sec.	air	variable to 1000	50, 100, 200, 400	.02, .05, .1, .2, paint	SL via articulating arm
Coherent Radiation	continuous wave	water	variable to more than 2000	50, 100, 200, 500 & 1000	0.2, .02, .05, .1, .2, .5, 1, 2, 5, continuous	SL and direct via articulating arm
Lynex	pulsed 3000/sec.	air	variable to 1000	altered from to 50 to 250	.05, .1, .25	SL & monocular indirect via fiber optic cable
MIRA	continuous wave	water	variable to 550 at 4880 Å 650 at 5145 Å	50, 100, 150, 250, & 500 with micro-scope variable to 1000 with monocular indirect	.05, .1, .2, .3, .5, .8, 1.0, 2.5 sec.	operating micro-scope & monocular indirect via articulating arm
O.T.I.	continuous wave	water	variable at 50 to at least 350 & at 200 to at least 500	50, 100, 200	selectable range of .05 to continuous	SL, direct and monocular indirect via fiber optic cable

Data compiled from advertisements from the respective companies.

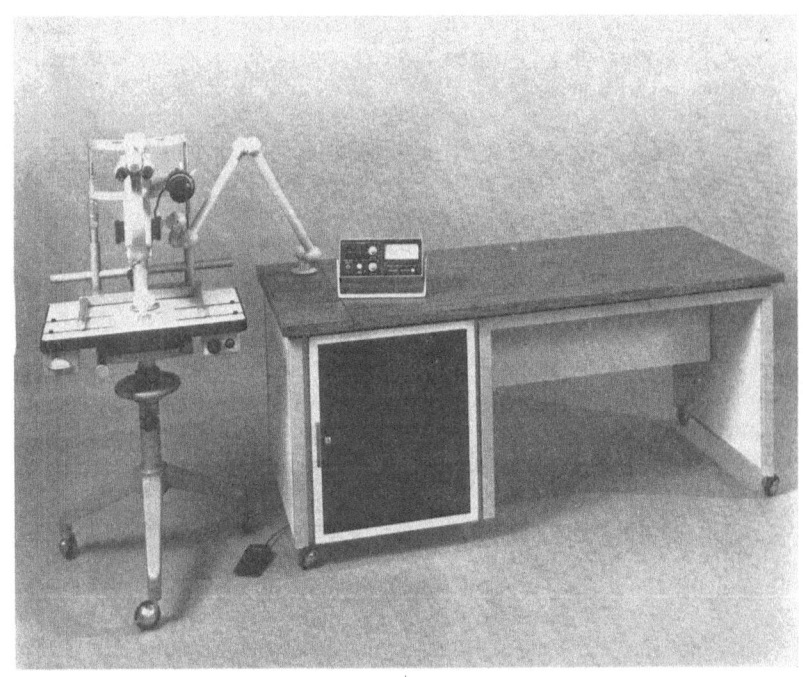

Fig. 1. Coherent Radiation argon laser slit lamp photocoagulator.

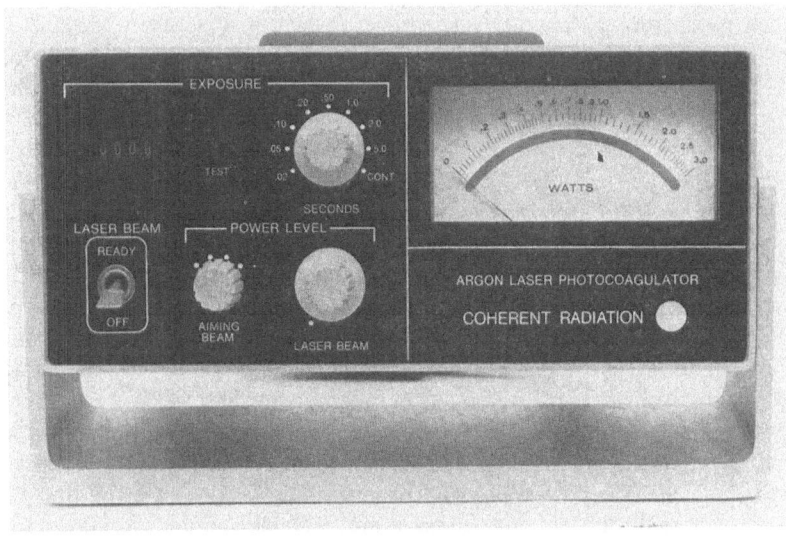

Fig. 2. Control panel indicating number of exposures, time in seconds, and power in watts.

not the purpose of this paper. The various argon laser photocoagulators are subject to developmental changes. Since most of the instruments have not stood the test of time, detailed evaluations cannot be given. In the selection of an instrument, information should be requested concerning safety features and photocoagulation parameters of the instrument, reliability and service of the company, and laboratory and clinical data to assure the surgeon that the instrument is dependable. Since the author's experience has been restricted to the Coherent Radiation slit lamp argon laser photocoagulator, the remainder of the discussion will be restricted to instrumentation of this photocoagulator and to the techniques in treatment of patients.

The argon laser used is a continuous wave 4 watt ion laser. It is housed within a desk-like cabinet in which there is also a compartment for the power source of the laser (Fig. 1). On the surface of the desk is situated a moveable control panel (Fig. 2) on which the power is monitored ranging from 0 to 3000 milliwatts. The time can be adjusted from 0.02 seconds to continuous wave application. For the most part applications are placed from .1 to .5 second duration. A knob is available to increase the intensity of the aiming light which is an attenuated portion of the argon beam below damage threshold of the human eye. There is an automatic counter to note the number of coagulations. The safety switch is turned on only at the moment the operator is ready to begin treatment. The laser beam passes through the articulating arm into the slit lamp delivery system. The Zeiss slit lamp system is constructed in a manner that the beam passes through one of a series of lenses that change the retinal spot size from 50, 100, 200, 500, and 1000 microns in size. In the American Optical slit lamp delivery system, a zoom lens is used to enable the operator to vary the size anywhere between 50 and 1000 microns in diameter. The beam then passes through another spherical lens which is attached to the micromanipulator. The operator by moving the handle of the micromanipulator alters by prismatic displacement the position of the laser independent of the viewing field. The beam then continues through a hole within the center of a mirror which reflects the illuminating light of the slit lamp. The hole bored through the center of this mirror enables the argon beam to be coaxial with the illuminating light of the slit lamp. The beam then enters the eye by way of a contact lens to correct any ametropia of the eye. The current argon laser photocoagulator has a power output up to 2000 milliwatts available to the eye. The available control panel indicates power up to 2000 milliwatts. For previous models an additional monitor to calibrate powers greater than 1000 milliwatts can be attached. For brighter illumination the light source of the Zeiss photo slit lamp can be changed from a 30 to 50 watt bulb. This requires a different power supply for the light. Zeiss provides an observer tube which can be attached to the photo slit lamp in order to facilitate other personnel to observe the operator in the process of photocoagulation.

A number of different contact lenses are available and are satisfactory for argon laser slit lamp photocoagulation. These include the Goldmann macular contact lens for treating lesions in the posterior pole, the Goldmann three mirror contact lens for treating lesions in the peripheral retina, the Lovac contact lenses, and various other contact lenses of similar nature. Such lenses should have a special antireflection coating to reduce the intensity of the argon laser beam reflected from the surface of the contact lens.

All patients require a complete ophthalmological examination before treatment. Such an examination should require accurate retinal drawings and preoperative photography. The photography of cases with macular diseases should show a fixation target in order for the operator to know where the patient is fixing, preventing treatment in this area. Another method to identify fixation is to have the patient fixate on the argon aiming beam before treatment. With this information one can avoid coagulating the patient's point of retinal fixation.

With the exception of patients being treated for retinal tears, fluorescein angiography is indispensible in the preoperative work-up. Fluorescein angiograms are necessary for the localization of macular leaks in central serous retinopathy, senile choroidal macular degeneration, and histoplasmic choroiditis. In diabetes and branch vein occlusions with vascular leakage into the macula, fluorescein angiography aids in the localization of areas requiring treatment. In the treatment of proliferative neovascular processes, early arterial phase angiograms aid in the detection of feeder vessels to neovascular fronds. The appropriate angiograms are selected and enlarged for better visualization of areas to be treated. At the time of treatment the enlarged photographs are placed adjacent to the operator for viewing. Dr. ARNOLD PATZ of Baltimore, Maryland, first recommended this technique. He further suggested

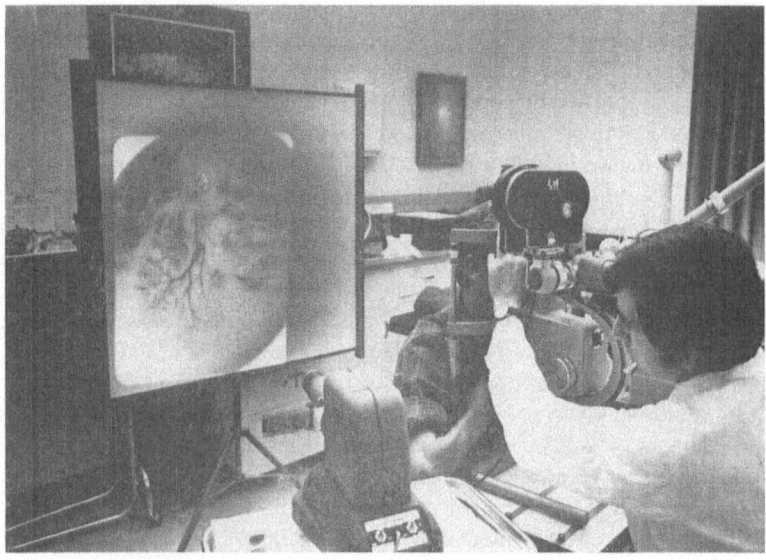

Fig. 3. Projected image of fluorescein angiographic negative provides enlarged view of feeder vessel. Fluorescein appears black in the negative.

the projection of the fluorescein negatives onto a screen as another method of studying enlargements of the vessels to be treated (Fig. 3). Of course when the negatives are projected the vessels containing fluorescein are black.

The use of retrobulbar injections is seldom necessary in the course of argon laser photocoagulation. With extreme photophobia and in rare cases of the very anxious patient with a juxtafoveal lesion, retrobulbar injection is required. Occasionally when treating feeder vessels that are entwined within a mesh of other vessels, one sometimes needs to use retrobulbar injection. Retrobulbar injections are necessary in less than 5 % of the cases treated.

There are three important components in any form of photocoagulation: the light source, the delivery system, and the operator. With argon laser energy, the wavelength of light is optimal for treating vascular disorders and for stimulating retinal pigment epithelial scars. With the slit lamp delivery system there is high magnification, good illumination and stereopsis for viewing the fundus. The operator is the all important third component in the process. He must be familiar with disease processes under treatment, adept at interpreting fluorescein angiograms, and knowledgeable in the process of laser photo-coagulation.

In discussing argon laser photocoagulation therapy, the following four parameters are involved: power measured in milliwatts, spot size measured in microns, time measured in seconds or fractions thereof, and number of lesions applied. In order to make objective evaluations of the effect of coagulation and in order to correlate the treatment with specific results, accurate data must be tabulated with each treatment.

It is important to have an accurate description of the retina under treatment and when possible a specific diagnosis should be made. Preoperative and postoperative evaluations of visual acuity, clinical appearance, and intravenous fluorescein angiograms are necessary to objectively evaluate the results.

The actual process of photocoagulation should be made with the operator in a relaxed position while the slit lamp is fixed in a position where the area under treatment is in full view. With the index finger on the micromanipulator and with the other hand on the contact lens, the operator is ready to procede with photocoagulation (Fig. 4). The exact power setting, spot size and time settings are best learned with experience. However, for 0.1 of a second exposure time, the following settings are usually satisfactory: 50 micron spot with 75 milliwatts of power, 100 micron spot with 100 milliwatts of power, 200 micron spot with 200 milliwatts of power, 500 micron spot with 400 milliwatts of power, and 1000 micron spot 700 to 1000 milliwatts of power.

In discussing power settings it is important to note that the intensity of the coagulation point varies for the same settings in treating different areas of the retina. Because of greater pigmentation in the macula, settings that give a rather light lesion in the paramacular region will produce a moderately heavy lesion in the parafoveal area (Fig. 5). Furthermore, lesions produced with similar settings in the far periphery are heavier than those in the midperiphery. In treating a more heavily pigmented region, the power likewise must be reduced. With the same spot size setting, a lesion produced with higher power

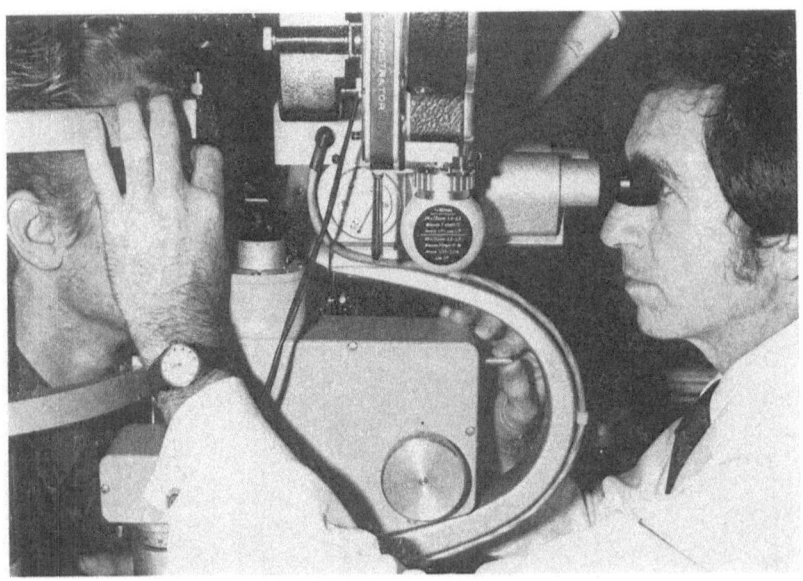

Fig. 4. With slit lamp in fixed position, the photocoagulator holds contact lens with one hand and the micromanipulator with the other hand.

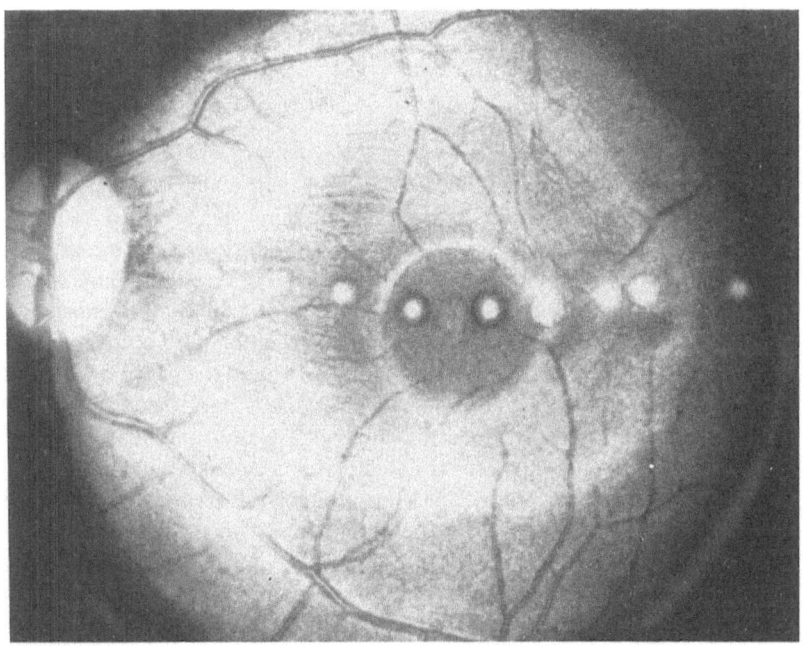

Fig. 5. Note heavier parafoveal lesions produced in Rhesus monkey with same power, time, and spot size settings.

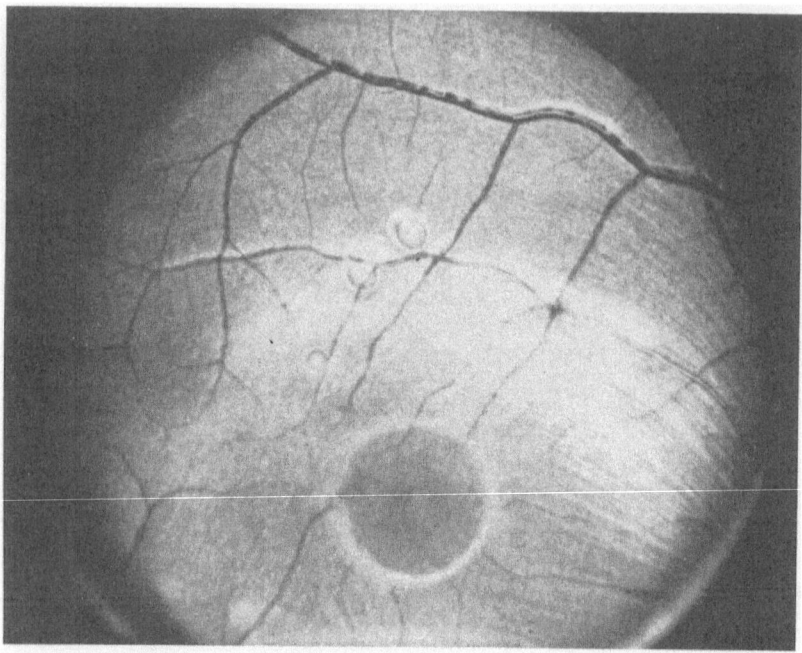

Fig. 6. The diameter of lesions produced in Rhesus monkey increases with increase of power settings without changing spot size or exposure time settings. All lesions produced with 50 micron diameter setting.

will be larger than one produced with a lower power. A 50 micron spot with 200 milliwatts of power at 0.1 of a second will be larger than a 50 micron spot produced at 50 milliwatts of power at 0.1 of a second (Fig. 6). Also for similar spot size and power settings, a lesion produced with a longer time exposure will be larger than a lesion produced with a minimal time setting. Thus, a lesion produced with a 50 micron spot at 1.0 second and 100 milliwatts of power will be larger than one produced by a 50 micron spot at 0.1 of a second and 100 milliwatts of power. If the diameter of a lesion is reduced to one half the original diameter, the area of the lesion is actually ¼th the area of the original lesion due to the law of πr^2. Therefore, the number of photons impinged upon the smaller spot assuming the power is not changed is actually four times greater on the smaller spot than on the larger one. It is mandatory that one reduce the power of the laser when one reduces the spot size. If this is not done, hemorrhage is likely to occur.

Since the wavelength of the argon laser beam activates fluorescein, intravenous fluorescein can be given immediately before treatment. This procedure assists in the localization of leaking areas during the time of treatment. Fluorescein pooled beneath retinal pigment epithelial elevations and within microaneurysms is easily identified at the time of treatment. By this technique microaneurysms can be differentiated from blot and dot hemorrhages. This facilitates in the treatment of macular lesions. It is used in addition to fluorescein photography; it is not a substitute for fluorescein photography.

With rare exceptions all cases are treated as outpatients. The postoperative care is quiet activity for three weeks, head elevation day and night to minimize elevations of venous pressure in the eye, and the use of pinhole glasses in some instances. Patients are instructed to avoid any situation that would involve a valsalva type maneuver as might occur with lifting, constipation, or sexual intercourse.

The patients are instructed to return for follow-up visits the day after treatment; if vessels have reopened subsequent treatment is carried out immediately. For most macular lesions no subsequent treatment is performed for three weeks to await results of the initial treatment. Following three to four weeks, repeat fluorescein angiography is carried out. If a leak is still present subsequent treatment is given. In cases of diabetic retinopathy, follow-up evaluation is advised at four week intervals until the disease process is brought under reasonable control with the fundus picture being quiescent. Once this is achieved, the patients are followed every three to four months with repeat dilated fundus examinations and fluorescein studies. Fluorescein angioscopy, a technique of giving fluorescein intravenously and studying the fundus with indirect ophthalmoscopy or slit lamp biomicroscopy with a cobalt filter between the viewing light and the retina enables the observer to detect any new pathologic areas since they readily fluoresce. If such areas are detected, appropriate fluorescein angiograms and enlargements are obtained to identify vessels requiring further treatment.

The technique of argon laser retinal photocoagulation is a subspecialty within ophthalmology. The operator must be well informed in retinal diseases and their treatment, in fluorescein angiography, and in techniques of laser photocoagulation. Since the field has undergone tremendous changes within the past three years, and since long term follow-up results have not yet been obtained, the patients are instructed that the techniques are still to be considered in the investigative stage. In cases of symmetrical retinopathy it is suggested that the operator treat only one eye, at least until the treated eye is considered a success with the retinal disease process quiescent. A three to six months lapse is recommended before treating the second eye.

A brief comment will be made about complications. The most significant complication in argon laser photocoagulation is hemorrhage (LITTLE & ZWENG, 1971). This usually occurs as a result of using too much power with small spot size settings. It is likely to occur if one coagulates efferent vessels leading from a frond, thus producing venous engorgement and hemorrhage. One is cautioned not to use powers over 300 and 400 milliwatts with spot sizes of 50 and 100 microns. Further discussion on complications will be given in another paper.

REFERENCES

LITTLE, H. L., ZWENG, H. C. & PEABODY, R. R.: Argon laser slitlamp retinal photocoagulation. *Trans. Amer. Acad. Ophthal. Otolaryng.* 74: *85–97* (1970).

LITLE, H. L. & ZWENG, H. C.: Complications of argon laser retinal photocoagulation. *Trans. Pac. Coast Oto-ophthal. Soc.* 52: *115–129* (1971).

PATZ, A.: Personal communication.

Key Words:
Argon laser retinal photocoagulation
Instrumentation
Techniques
Fluorescein angiography
Fluorescein angioscopy

COMPARISON BETWEEN
LASER-PHOTOCOAGULATION AND
XENON-PHOTOCOAGULATION

G. MEYER-SCHWICKERATH

(*Essen*)

Since 6 years we have experience with different types of rubin-lasers. We have used the instrument of KEELER and were not content with it. The threshold between a normal clinical reaction and overdosage is very small so that explosive reactions with a hemorrhage or a gas-bubble in the centre are quite common.

A better instrument is the rubin-laser from AMERICAN OPTICAL which is by far more constant in the output of the laser energy. It remains however the same negative point that the coagulation time cannot be regulated. For this reason, if one moves from a place of low absorption to a place of high absorption, an explosive reaction may occur. From the clinical point of view it should be possible to regulate the coagulation time with the finger tip according to the reaction occuring in the retina. This is the safest technique to avoid overdosage.

My co-workers J. PESCH and O. E. LUND have reported our experimental and clinical observations in extenso.

Since almost 3 years we have a continuous argon-laser combined with the direct ophthalmoscope from the xenon-zeiss-photocoagulator. An additional light-source is used to give some visual field on the fundus. The light-beam of the argonlaser is spread to a diametre of 6 mm so that a coagulation of the iris or cornea may be avoided. In addition to this the light-beam can be diverged so that coagulations of the fundus can be produced from somewhat less than 50 microns up to 300. This instrument has the advantage that it can be used by regulating the coagulation time with the finger tip as with the old xenon-coagulator. On the other hand in several indications we have been rather disappointed because of several disadvantages.

By using a very small coagulation spot it is difficult to set the correct dosage. A very small change in the output energy can result suddenly in overtreatment. This is in contrast to larger coagulations.

On the other hand, if we want to perform a larger coagulation in the retinal periphery, we found it rather difficult because the energy has to be brought up to almost 1000 mW. Under these circumstances retrobulbar injection might be necessary so that one of the great advantages, Dr. LITTLE has discussed, disappears. For example, if we want to seal off a peripheral retinal tear with small argon-photocoagulations we have to use several hundred individual coagulations which is a very time-taking procedure. We also found it difficult

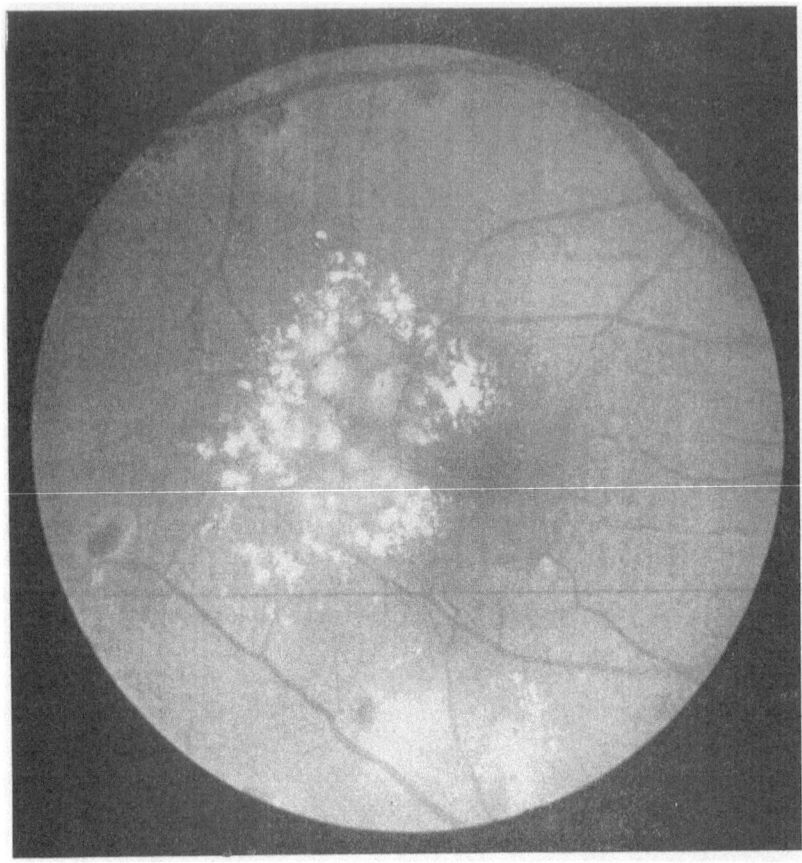

Fig. 1. Leber's microaneurysm retinitis. The small aneurysms have been treated with 100 mikron argoncoagulations. In the periphery xenoncoagulations of 3 degrees, 2 months old.

to coagulate edematous retina as well as very flat detachments, because they occur frequently in the vicinity of peripheral holes. In contrast to xenon-coagulation this is probably only because of the size of the coagulation field. In the histopathological pictures we can see that a typical argon-coagulation has very steep edges whereas xenon-photocoagulation has smooth edges.

We did not have good reactions in intraocular tumours as angiomatosis retinae, retinoblastoma and malignant melanoblastoma. The same is true for most cases of Eales' disease and Coats' disease and of diabetic retinopathy which will be discussed later.

The argon-photocoagulator is however very useful if we want to destroy small areas in the vicinity of the disc and the macula. Several slides are shown in which small aneurysms, some due to Leber's microaneurysm-retinitis, could be destroyed in the immediate vicinity of the macula without damaging valuable tissue. The same is true for diabetic retinopathy which will be discussed later.

Our experience with the argon-photocoagulator is that it is a very useful instrument to destroy small areas at the posterior pole. For most other indications the xenon-coagulation is either quicker or easier or safer in the way we use it. We have however not yet the instrument which can be used in connection with the slit lamp.

We are using photocoagulation to seal off retinal tears in most of our cases at the end of detachment operations or a few days later. This is an indication in which xenon-coagulation on the patient under general anesthesia seems to be superior.

PREOPERATIVE EVALUATION OF
MACULAR ALTERATIONS,
FLUORESCEIN STUDIES

A. WESSING

(Essen)

Fluorescein angiography is undoubtedly one of the most important preconditions for the diagnosis and treatment of macular diseases. The combination of angiographic examination and photocoagulation offers a broad variety of possibilities for a successful therapy of exudative maculopathies.

I will try to demonstrate the most important disease entities and their angiographic symptoms. The importance of ophthalmoscopy and biomicroscopy with the contact glas and the different tests of function shall, of course, not be neglected.

I. CENTRAL SEROUS RETINOPATHY

At first there is central serous retinal detachment with the wellknown circumscribed fluorescein leakage spots. They are the aim for photocoagulation especially in those cases where no spontaneous improvement occurs within 4 to 6 weeks and where secondary degenerations of the detached retina develop.

I should mention that central serous retinal detachment may progress to a generalized exudative detachment of the whole retina. It ends up in a picture which corresponds to Harada's disease. Fluorescein angiography shows multiple areas of severe dye leakage. Such an extreme progression seems to be rare, but at the fluorescein symposium in Tokyo about ten cases have been presented.

2. CENTRAL HEMORRHAGIC RETINAL DETACHMENT

Fluorescein angiography shows that the origin of subretinal idiopathic hemorrhages is closely related to the simple subretinal serous exudate and that the difference is only of quantitative nature. In some cases fluorescein leakage may be found. Usually, however, the hemorrhage is hiding the view to the choroid and to the leakage points. But as this type of maculopathy is progressive we think coagulation might be indicated, even if the source of the hemorrhages is not visible.

3. CHOROIDAL VASCULAR PROLIFERATION

Vessel proliferation from the choroid into the subretinal space have rarely been described. They are quite frequently in focal choroiditis or so-called histoplasmosis, but they can also be found in other hemorrhagic macular diseases.

In the arterial phase fluorescein angiography shows a clearly outlined subretinal vascular pattern without connections to the retinal vessels. But already in the early venous phase dye leakage starts and some seconds later the complete area is covered by extravascular dye. As a rule the new formed vessels are hidden by the pigment epithelium or blood and can be detected only with the aid of fluorescein angiography. They practically always give rise to recurrent subretinal hemorrhages with tremendous damage to central vision. Photocoagulation treatment therefore should be attempted, even if the lesions are situated in the macular area.

4. MACULOPATHY IN GRÖNBLAD-STRANDBERG'S SYNDROME

When angoid streaks reach the macular area there usually develops a severe maculopathy. By fluorescein angiography it very often is possible to find the sources of the subretinal hemorrhages and exudates. The breaks in Bruch's membrane and the defects in the pigment epithelium are very well outlined and the spots of dye leakage can be localized for photocoagulation.

5. TRAUMATIC MACULOPATHY

Months or years after traumatic choroidal ruptures there may develop hemorrhagic or exudative maculopathy. In most of these cases fluorescein injection reveales areas of dye leakage adjacent to the choroidal ruptures which can be coagulated.

6. FUCHS' SPOT

Very similar conditions are found in highly myopic eyes with Fuchs' spot: hemorrhages, ruptures in the pigment epithelium and Bruch's membrane, and sometimes subretinal vascular proliferations from the choroid too.

7. DETACHMENT OF THE PIGMENT EPITHELIUM

In contrast to the central serous maculopathy the detachment of the pigment-epithelium is characterized by an overall staining and the absence of real leakage spots. Photocoagulation therefore will be difficult or even impossible and ineffective.

8. SENILE SCLEROTIC MACULOPATHY

As we learned from fluorescein angiography there are close relationships between senile maculopathy and detachment of the pigment epithelium. Extensive detachment of the pigment epithelium may lead to a more or less typical macular degeneration after many years. On the other hand many cases of Junius-Kuhnt's disease are combined with extensive detachment of the pigment epithelium.

A statistical evaluation of 35 cases of pigment epithelial detachment out of our own material confirms these close relations. Younger patients between 35 and 45 years of age usually showed a spontaneous improvement. Patients beyond the fifth decade developed severe loss of central vision after 2 to 3 years.

Besides detachment of the pigment epithelium a few cases show circumscribed leakage spots. This however, holds true only in the very early stage of the disease. Other cases develop subretinal vascular proliferation from the choriocapillaris.

In our experience the results of photocoagulation in senile maculopathy are not very convincing. The only exception are those cases with leakage spots or vascular proliferation. A thorough search for these cases is therefore important.

SUMMARY

Fluorescein angiographic symptoms of exudative macular lesions are described and the indications for photocoagulation are outlined.

REFERENCES

GASS, J. D. M.: Stereoscopic atlas of macular diseases. Mosby St. Louis (1970).
WESSING, A.: Photocoagulation in the treatment of macular lesions. *Acta Congr. Ophthal.* 19: *507–508* (Mexico, 1970).

MACULAR DISEASES: CLASSIFICATION AND TREATMENT WITH ARGON LASER SLIT LAMP PHOTOCOAGULATION

HUNTER L. LITTLE, M.D.

(Palo Alto, California)

Clarification of nomenclature and of macular disease syndromes is essential before discussing photocoagulation of macular diseases. The classification of macular diseases can be based on the pathology as visualized during ophthalmological examination and on histopathologic examination of specimens submitted to the laboratory (GASS, 1967; MAUMENEE, 1965; ZWENG et al., 1969). Distinction of the terms retinal detachment, retinal edema, and retinal cysts is required. Retinal detachment is a separation of the retina from the underlying structures by accumulation of subretinal serous or hemorrhagic fluid or by inflammatory, reactive hyperplastic, or neoplastic cells (GASS, 1967). The separation can be between the retinal pigment epithelium and Bruch's membrane (a retinal pigment epithelial detachment), between the retinal pigment epithelium and the sensory retina (a detachment of the sensory retina), or between both the retinal pigment epithelium and Bruch's membrane and the retinal pigment epithelium sensory retina. The detached sensory retina is usually semitransparent and normal in thickness without edema; however, with prolonged elevation of the sensory retina, it undergoes edematous changes and cystic degeneration.

Retinal edema is the accumulation of fluid within the retina. The accumulated fluid can be intracellular manifested in central retinal artery occlusion where cell death is associated with cell swelling. It can be extracellular from capillary effusion within the retina manifested by retinal vein thrombosis, diabetic retinopathy, hypertensive retinopathy, and cystoid macular edema in aphakia. In both kinds of edema the retinal thickness is increased and the retinal transparency is decreased. The following descriptive classification of macular diseases is presented to summarize the above statements (Table I).

Retinal cysts are sac-like distensions within one of the plexiform layers of the sensory retina. Retinal cysts are an exaggerated form of extracellular retinal edema. There is progressive distension within the plexiform layers and obliteration of the adjacent tissues. If the inner wall of the cyst ruptures, there is an apparent retinal hole. Since the hole involves only the inner layer of the sensory retina, a rhegmatogenous retinal detachment with accumulation of fluid between the sensory retina and the retinal pigment epithelium cannot occur until the hole extends through all layers of the sensory retina. Excepting in

Palo Alto Medical Clinic, Palo Alto Medical Research Foundation and Stanford University School of Medicine, Palo Alto, California.

Table I. *Descriptive Classification of Macular Lesions.*

1. Detachment of sensory retina
   a. serous
   b. hemorrhagic
2. Detachment of retinal pigment epithelium
   a. serous
   b. hemorrhagic
3. Edema
   a. intracellular — retinal artery occlusion
   b. extracellular — cystoid macular edema
      1. vein occlusion
      2. diabetes
      3. hypertension
      4. aphakia

macular holes with trauma and in high myopia, macular holes are usually lamellar and incomplete, thus not necessitating treatment with photocoagulation.

Central serous choroidopathy (retinopathy) is an example of a localized serous detachment of the retinal pigment epithelium with a larger overlying serous detachment of the sensory retina within the macula. Senile choroidal macular degeneration can present in a similar manner; however, the choroidal leaks are usually more diffuse and more numerous. The leaks are frequently associated with underlying choroidal neovascularization extending through breaks in Bruch's membrane beneath the retinal pigment epithelium and with resultant hemorrhagic detachments of the retinal pigment epithelium. Similar findings occur in histoplasmic choroiditis within the macula. In contrast to serous detachments of the retinal pigment epithelium which have a light fawn color and which are translucent thus not obscuring underlying fluorescence on angiography, hemorrhagic detachments of the retinal pigment epithelium have a slight grey appearance suggestive of a choroidal melanoma and a faint red halo surrounding the margin of the hemorrhagic pigment epithelial detachment. Hemorrhagic detachments of the retinal pigment epithelium are not translucent, thus block activation of underlying fluorescein. Hemorrhagic detachments of the retinal pigment epithelium may undergo organization with subsequent development of a disciform white scar. Such lesions result in permanent loss of central vision.

In addition to a descriptive classification of macular diseases, an etiologic classification of macular diseases is essential (Table II). The organization of such a classification is subject to criticism and is certain to change as future knowledge is gained in the understanding of the pathologic physiology of macular diseases. Broad headings of degenerative disorders, inflammatory disorders, metabolic disorders, neoplastic disorders, traumatic disorders, toxic disorders, and congenital anomalies are listed. It is debatable whether diabetic retinopathy with its vascular changes should be included under metabolic diseases or under degenerative diseases. The various heredomacular

Table II. *Etiologic Classification of Macular Diseases.*

1. Degenerative
   a. central serous choroidopathy (retinopathy)
   b. senile choroidal macular degeneration
   c. retinal vascular disease (diabetes and hypertension)
2. Inflammatory
   a. histoplasmic choroiditis
   b. histoplasmic like choroiditis
   c. toxoplasmosis retinochoroiditis
   d. toxocara canis ocular infestation
   e. solar retinitis (foveomacular retinitis)
   f. preretinal membrane contracture
   g. acute multifocal posterior placoid pigment epitheliopathy (AMPPPE)
3. Metabolic
   a. heredomacular degenerations (vitelliform, Stargardt's, flavimaculatus, etc.)
   b. tapetoretinal degenerations (retinitis pigmentosa)
   c. cerebromacular degeneration (Tay-Sachs's and Niemann-Pieck's)
4. Neoplastic
   a. nevus
   b. malignant melanoma
   c. choroidal hemangioma
   d. metastatic
5. Traumatic
6. Toxic maculopathies
7. Congenital anomalies

diseases including vitelliform macular degeneration, Stargardt's macular degeneration, flavimaculatus, and retinitis pigmentosa are included under metabolic disorders. Nonetheless, the ophthalmologist when viewing the macula is urged to make an accurate description of the macular syndrome in question and to make an attempt to categorize the syndrome into one of the above mentioned etiologic groups. Grouping aids in the evaluation of the natural course and in the response of treatment.

Table III. *Criteria for Selection of Macular Lesions. Amenable to Photocoagulation.*

1. Presence of fluid (serous or hemorrhagic) with localized leakage demonstrable with fluorescein angiography
   a. intraretinal — edema
   b. subretinal — beneath sensory retina
   c. subretinal pigment epithelium
2. Neovascularization
   a. retinal
   b. choroidal
Treatment of foveal leakage is usually contraindicated

Table IV. *Macular Diseases Amenable to Argon Laser Photo-coagulation.*

---

1. Central serous choroidopathy (retinopathy)
3. Senile choroidal macular degeneration
3. Histoplasmic choroiditis
4. Macular edema
   a. diabetic retinopathy
   b. branch vein occlusion
   c. cystoid macular edema (rarely)

Table III lists the criteria in the selection of macular lesions amenable to treatment with photocoagulation. These criteria include the presence of serous or hemorrhagic fluid within the retina, beneath the sensory retina, or beneath the retinal pigment epithelium with demonstrable leak on fluorescein angiography; the presence of retinal or choroidal neovascularization. Treatment of foveal leakage is usually contraindicated. In all cases the question should be asked as to whether the natural course of the disease or the scar produced by photocoagulation will produce the greater visual impairment.

Table IV lists the macular syndromes amenable to photocoagulation (Table IV). These include central serous choroidopathy, senile choroidal macular degeneration, histoplasmic choroiditis, and macular edema associated with diabetic retinopathy and branch vein occlusion.

TECHNIQUE

Preoperative evaluation includes a complete ophthalmological examination including best corrected visual acuity, central visual fields including the Amsler grid and detailed funduscopic examination with the contact lens at the slit lamp. Intravenous fluorescein angiographic studies of the macula using 5 cc of 10% fluorescein are essential. The fluorescein photographs are taken with a fundus camera using the Baird atomic B4 filter between the light source and the retina and a Baird atomic B5 filter between the film and the retina. Tri-X Pan film with an ASA value of 400 is used. Enlargements of the pictures provide greater detail of the area to be treated. In addition, stereo photographs assist in determining whether the leak is retinal or choroidal in origin. Leaks are identified by blurring of the margins of the area of fluorescein and by persistence of the fluorescence on 45 minute delayed pictures. Polaroid photographs are taken showing the fixation target in order to determine the location of the leak in relation to the point of fixation. The fixation target should also be used on the fluorescein studies to identify the relationship of the area of fluorescence with the point of fixation.

The patient is seated before the argon slit lamp photocoagulator. Immediately prior to treatment another intravenous injection may be given to assist in the localization of the leaking area during the time of argon laser photo-

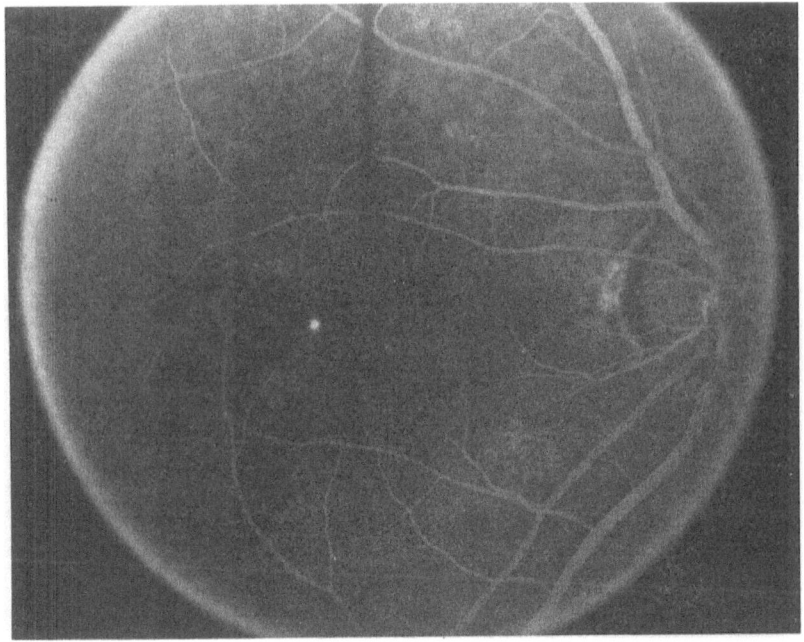

Fig. 1. Pretreatment fluorescein angiogram in central serous choroidopathy (retinopathy) shows discrete leak.

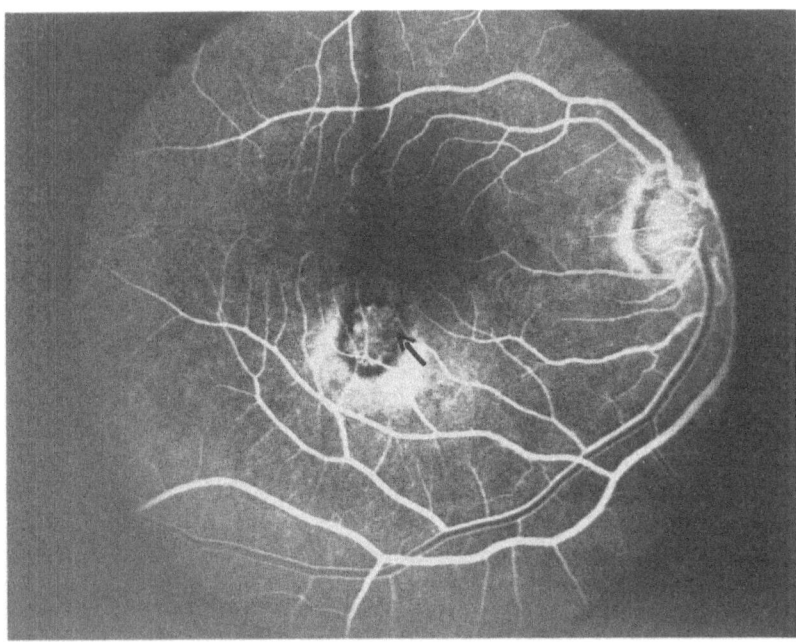

Fig. 2. Pretreatment fluorescein angiogram reveals choroidal neovascularization in histoplasmic choroiditis.

coagulation. For lesions of the posterior pole, the macular Goldmann contact lens is used.

The usual settings in the treatment of small areas of leakage in central serous choroidopathy (Fig. 1) are as follows: 100 micron spot size, .05 or .1 second exposure time, and 75 to 125 milliwatts. The end point of coagulation should be a mild blanching of the retinal pigment epithelium in the area of fluorescein leakage. In cases with large pigment epithelial detachment, greater power is necessary to obliterate the leakage. The setting for such cases usually requires a 100 or 200 micron spot size with .1 to .2 second exposure time, and 150 to 300 milliwatts. For cases in which one demonstrates underlying choroidal neovascularization as occurs in senile choroidal macular degeneration and histoplasmic choroidopathy (Fig. 2), moderately heavy lesions are necessary to obliterate the leaking vessels (Fig. 3, 4). Minimal coagulation in such cases frequently results in hemorrhage and/or increased choroidal neovascularization. The usual settings for this kind of lesion are as follows: 200 to 500 micron spot size, .2 second exposure time, and 200 to 500 milliwatts power. The end point of coagulation is a densely white area covering the entire leakage point. When space permits, one usually places a barrage of coagulation between the lesion and the fovea. Such a barrier is placed with a 50 to 100 micron spot, .05 to .1 second, and 75 to 100 milliwatts. This arc of coagulation is placed in an attempt to prevent the extension of hemorrhage from the lesion into the fovea.

Sixty five eyes have been treated for central serous retinopathy. All have improved subsequent to argon laser photocoagulation. Several of the central serous retinopathy cases required two to three treatment sessions before clearing.

The results of the senile choroidal macular degeneration group were discouraging since new leaks frequently occurred after sealing old leaks. Visual acuity may not improve for 6 to 12 months after the leaks are sealed and after the localized retinal detachment has been flattened. One third of the eyes treated improved.

Fifty eyes with histoplasmic choroiditis were treated to determine the effect of argon laser photocoagulation on the course of this disease. All eyes in the study had visual impairment due to macular involvement. Critical evaluation of the results were made to determine what cases responded best to treatment.

Favorable responses occurred in eyes in which the margin of the lesion was greater than ¼ disc diameter from the fovea. Coupled with this qualification was pretreatment visual acuity of 20/50 or better. Favorable responses occurred in 60% of such cases only when moderately heavy argon laser photocoagulation was directed to the lesion. Serous detachment resolved; leaks on fluorescein angiography were significantly reduced or cleared; and final visual acuity remained 20/50 or better. Cases with vision worse than 20/50 usually had foveal involvement by the lesion or hemorrhage. Treatment was effective in less than 30% of such cases.

Criteria for improvement were visual acuity either improving or remaining the same, improvement of the clinical picture with clearing of serous detachment or hemorrhage, and reduction and usually absence of leakage on the fluorescein angiogram.

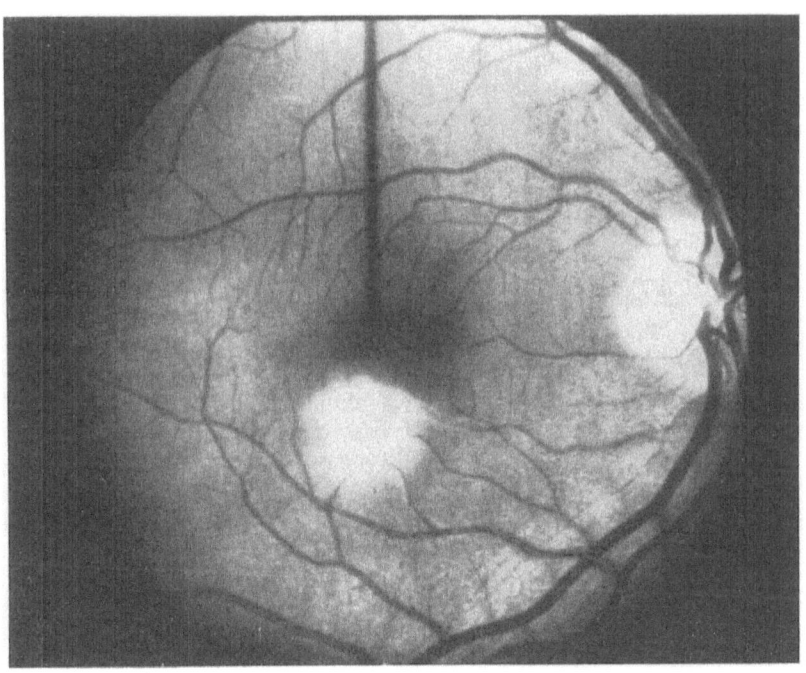

Fig. 3. Funduscopic appearance of intense photocoagulation lesion.

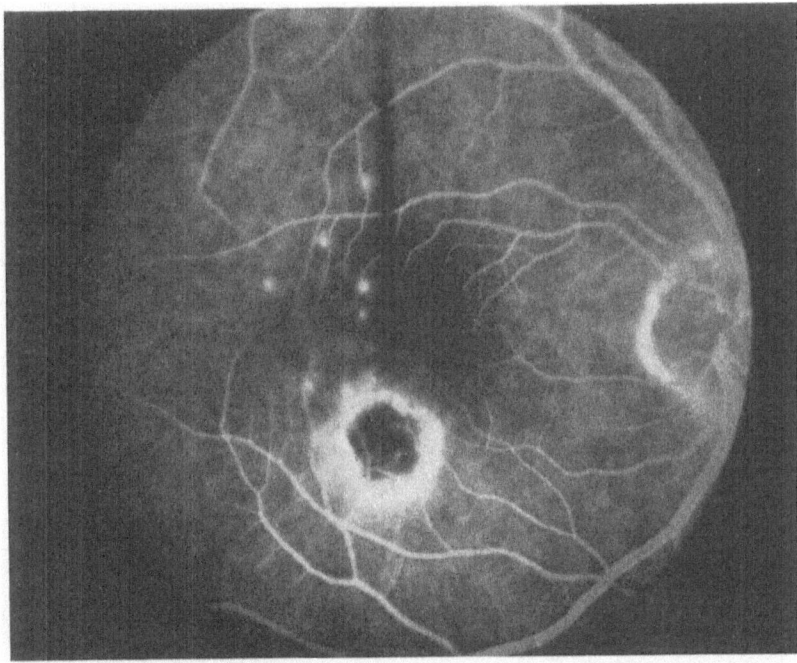

Fig. 4. Fluorescein angiogram four weeks after argon laser photocoagulation shows choroidal flush around margin of lesion with no residual choroidal neovascularization.

The following summary describes the results of treatment of various macular diseases by the author and Dr. H. C. ZWENG: 65 cases of central serous retinopathy were treated with clearing of serous detachment in all cases; 100 cases of senile choroidal macular degeneration were treated with improvement in 34%, no change in 28%, and progressive degeneration in 38%; and 50 cases of histoplasmic choroiditis showed 55% improved, 15% unchanged, and 30% worse. All cases included had follow-up periods ranging from 6 months to 3 years.

When indicated, argon laser photocoagulation is given to a miscellaneous group of macular entities associated with fluorescein leakage and presence of serous or hemorrhagic fluid beneath the pigment epithelium and the sensory retina. These include angioid streaks most frequently associated with pseudoxanthoma elasticum, macular degeneration in high myopia, and rare cases of congenital pit of the optic nerve with associated serous detachment of the sensory retina. The latter entity is usually not associated with the demonstration of a fluorescein leakage. It is only when such a point of leakage can be identified that treatment is indicated. Macular edema caused by branch retinal vein occlusion is sometimes amenable to photocoagulation.

SUMMARY

A descriptive and etiologic classification of macular diseases is given. Criteria for the selection of cases amenable to argon laser photocoagulation are listed, and the most common macular syndromes treatable by argon laser photocoagulation are given. Brief comment is made concerning techniques in preparation of patients for treatment and techniques involved with argon laser photocoagulation of macular diseases. A summary of the results following treatment is given.

REFERENCES

GASS, J. D. M.: Pathogenesis of disciform detachment of the neuroepithelium. I. General concepts and classification. *Amer. J. Ophthal.* 63: 573 (1967).
MAUMENEE, A. E.: Clinical manifestations. *Trans. Amer. Acad. Ophthal. Otolaryng.* 69: 605–613 (1965).
ZWENG, H. C., LITTLE, H. L. & PEABODY, R. R.: Laser Photocoagulation and Retinal Angiography. St. Louis, C. V. Mosby Co. (1969).

Key Words:
Argon laser slit lamp photocoagulation
Macular diseases
Indications for treatment
Macular edema
Detachment of retinal pigment epithelium
Detachment of sensory retina
Choroidal neovascularization
Central serous choroidopathy
Senile choroidal macular degeneration
Histoplasmic choroiditis
Fluorescein angiography

TECHNIQUES AND RESULTS OF PHOTOCOAGULATION IN NON DIABETIC VASCULAR DISEASES OF THE RETINA

A. WESSING

(*Essen*)

Eales' disease, Coats' disease or Leber's miliary aneurysm retinitis and v. Hippel's angiomatosis of the retina can be counted among the most important and rewarding indications for photocoagulation. Encouraged by reports from VERHOEFF, FRANCESCHETTI and WEVE on the favourable influence of diathermy coagulation MEYER-SCHWICKERATH started photocoagulation treatment of these three diseases in 1954. Our experience of about 20 years is mainly based on the use of the xenon arc photocoagulator. However, we have used the argon laser for three years. Especially tiny circumscribed lesions at the posterior pole lend themselves particularly for the smallest argon laser burns.

I. EALES' DISEASE

Technique of treatment

The technique of treatment was altered during the course of time. I shall describe it here in the manner in which it is carried out today (Fig. 1): All aneurysms and new-formed vessels must be coagulated. They are often only seen for the first time during photocoagulation. They become visible anterior to the whitish background of the coagulation. The vascular lesions are situated in the periphery of the retina especially in the early stages so that the resulting defect in the visual field is only small. Coagulation is simple enough if the vessels lie in the level of the retina and are not covered with exudate or hemorrhage. It is both dangerous and unnecessary to coagulate the dilated and curved feeding vessels. After coagulation of the peripheral lesions these vessels resume their normal structure and size.

In cases of vascular proliferation into the vitreous, one may try to close off the arterial and venous roots of these proliferations by coagulation at the basis.

The intensity of the photocoagulation used can be especially low in cases of Eales' disease. It is sufficient when, in $\frac{1}{2}$ sec, a fairly whitish discoloration of the retina occurs. The vessels themselves hardly change their appearance but in the course of 2–3 weeks one can recognize whether or not they are completely closed.

As a rule, we coagulate not more than one quarter of the retinal circumference. If larger regions in the periphery of the retina are affected, we leave an

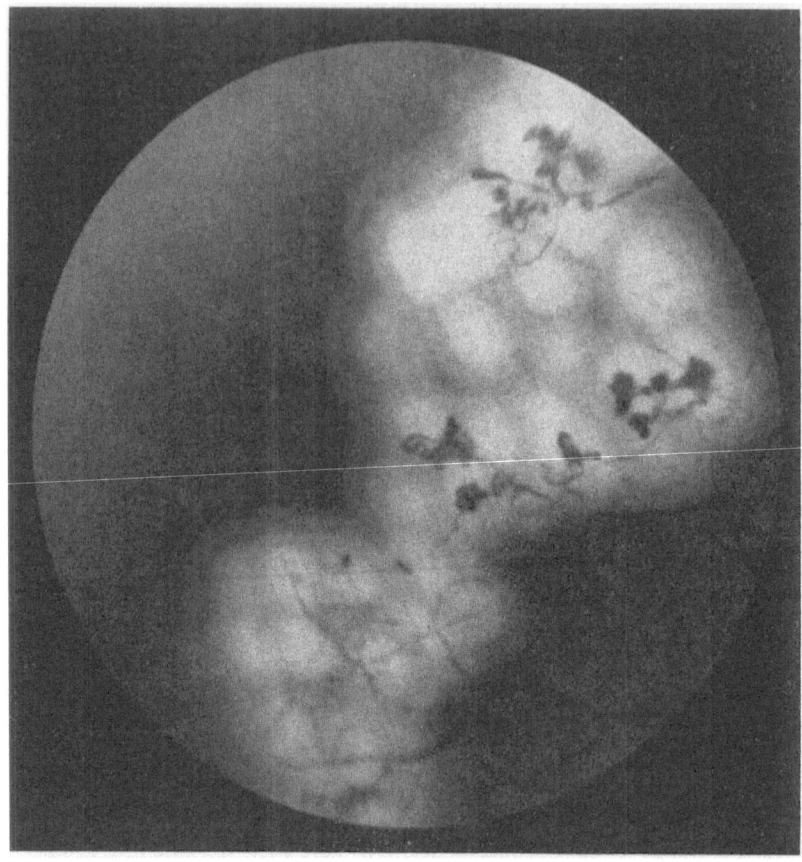

Fig. 1. Xenon arc coagulation in Eales' disease.

interval of 2 weeks between each coagulation treatment. The further course is marked by smooth avascular scars. The feeding vessels will be reduced to normal size. The scars are nearly always heavily pigmented. But months and years later they become more and more atrophic.

After the coagulation of all visible aneurysms has been carried out, follow-up examinations are made at intervals of 3 months. If new proliferations occur, these are treated again. They rarely develop in the region of old scars, but most often in untreated areas.

Results

Since 1954 we were able to follow the course of 143 treated eyes.

During a mean observation period of 3 years 124 (86%) eyes remained without further hemorrhage. Of these 124 symptom-free eyes only 7% showed

44

a decrease in visual acuity due to traction and exudative or degenerative processes in the region of the macula. The 14 % of treated eyes in which further symptoms occurred, were, on the whole, very severe and progressive cases with vascular lesions right in the centre of the fundus or with extensive proliferations into the vitreous.

Complications

The main complications of photo-coagulation in Eales' disease are hemorrhages, secondary retinal detachment and macular puckering.

To our own surprise, hemorrhages have proven to be a rare complication. Acute hemorrhages occurring during coagulation can mostly be stopped by immediate coagulation of the blood source. Small pre-retinal hemorrhages may occur one or two days after photocoagulation. They are due to the necrosis of the coagulated vessels and aneurysms and are normally reabsorbed within one or two weeks. Only one eye was lost by a severe irreversible vitreous hemorrhage.

Secondary detachment of the retina was observed in progressive cases with large vascular proliferations into the vitreous (9 cases = 7%). In more than half of the cases scleral infolding or cerclage operation were successfull and it was possible to complete the operation by coagulation of the aneurysms.

Postcoagulative macular puckering is the most dramatic and unfortunately a frequent complication in the treatment of Eales' disease.

Characteristically, there is an increased tortuosity of the smaller vessels in the macular area, with an alteration of their course. The surface of the involved retina has an increased shagreen or reflection with a crinkled cellophane-like appearance. Surprisingly, fluorescein usually does not leak from the affected vessels.

The process usually begins from a few weeks up to a few months, after photo-coagulation has been carried out. In most cases a permanent central scotoma remains. We observed these complications in about 4% of the treated cases. Postcoagulative maculopathy is the more serious since it concerned eyes with small lesions and good visual function.

Discussion

How can we explain the surprising effect of photo-coagulation in Eales' disease?

Eales' disease is up to now grouped under the inflammatory vascular disease of the retina (ASHTON). However the very early changes in the vascular pattern of the retina in Eales' disease do not show signs of inflammation (ELLIOT, MEYER-SCHWICKERATH). The concept of MEYER-SCHWICKERATH therefore is that Eales' disease is primarily not an inflammatory disease but an degenerative or occlusive one.

As already described by Eales this disease starts with changes in the extreme periphery of the fundus. It seems possible that the inital process is obliteration of the shunt-capillaries of the peripheral retina. This process, once set in motion, might become autonomous and then progress in a circulus vitiosus of ischemia and proliferation from the periphery to the centre. This circulus vitiosus would be interrupted by coagulation of the aneurysms and the new formed vessels.

Fluorescein angiography does confirm this hypothesis. The typical findings are obliterations of capillaries, arterioles and venules in the fundus periphery and capillary dilatation, microaneurysms and vessel proliferation on the edge of these avascular areas. There may develop a barrier of new formed vessels as a borderline of an avascular peripheral retina.

The most remarkable sign of all these pathological blood vessels is an impairment of permeability and one has to be aware that dye leakage is only an early step in the disturbance of the blood vessel's wall, which may end up with massive hemorrhages.

Inflammatory and degenerative lesions occur in later stages of the disease and should be considered as the result of hemodynamic disturbance.

The cause of the obliterating process up to now is unknown. But Eales' disease finds an interesting parallel in sickle-cell retinopathy. The retinal changes of this disease are ophthalmoscopically very similar to those found in Eales' disease and fluorescein angiography reveals the same symptoms: peripheral vascular obliteration with a barrier of new formed retinal vessels towards the centre. In sickle-cell disease we know that micro-embolisation leads to the occlusion of peripheral retinal capillaries. From this point of view it seems to be possible that a comparable process gives rise to Eales' disease.

II. COATS' DISEASE

Coats' disease and Leber's miliary aneurysm retinitis seem to be identical, congenital malformations of the retinal vascular system and they can be classified as retinal teleangiectasia (REESE). The early stages of the disease are characterized by severe changes of the capillary pattern. The normal capillaries are replaced by a rough network of dilated capillary channels. Different from diabetes or Eales' they show a straight course or they form large loops without changing in size. There are aneurysms which originate either from capillaries or from larger arterioles or venules. Fluorescein angiography shows very little or no dye leakage at all. In the later stages secondary changes may develop, as there are lipoidal deposits in the retina, intraretinal transsudation, hemorrhages and exudative detachment.

Technique of treatment

In the early stages treatment with photocoagulation is simple enough. All affected vessels are coagulated including main vascular branches and aneurysms (Fig. 2). Lipoidal deposits are not coagulated and they are not sealed off by a barrage of coagulation.

46

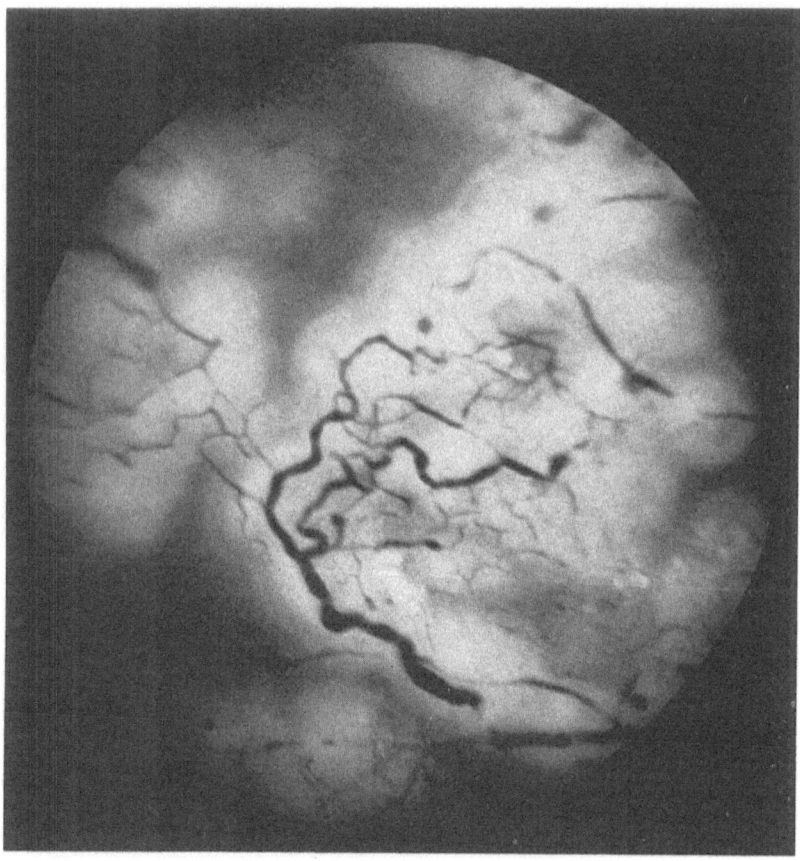

Fig. 2. Xenon arc coagulation in Coats' disease.

They reabsorbe and disappear spontaneously after destruction of all diseased vessels.

In advanced cases with intraretinal exudation and development of pseudo-tumours photocoagulation should be combined with epi- or intrascleral diathermy. In the case of exudative detachment coagulation may be combined with scleral infolding or any other buckling procedure.

An exception of these rules are circumscribed changes of the blood vessels which are confined to the macular area. Capillary dilatations near the macula are very often connected only with one single arteriole. Photocoagulation can aim either to occlude the main feeding vessel or to coagulate each aneurysm individually. One or two coagulations with the 1,5° field diaphragm may be sufficient to interrupt the blood flow in the feeding vessel and thereby to cut off the whole of the diseased capillary area. For coagulation of the aneurysms we prefer the argon laser. The aneurysms can easily be destroyed by the concen-

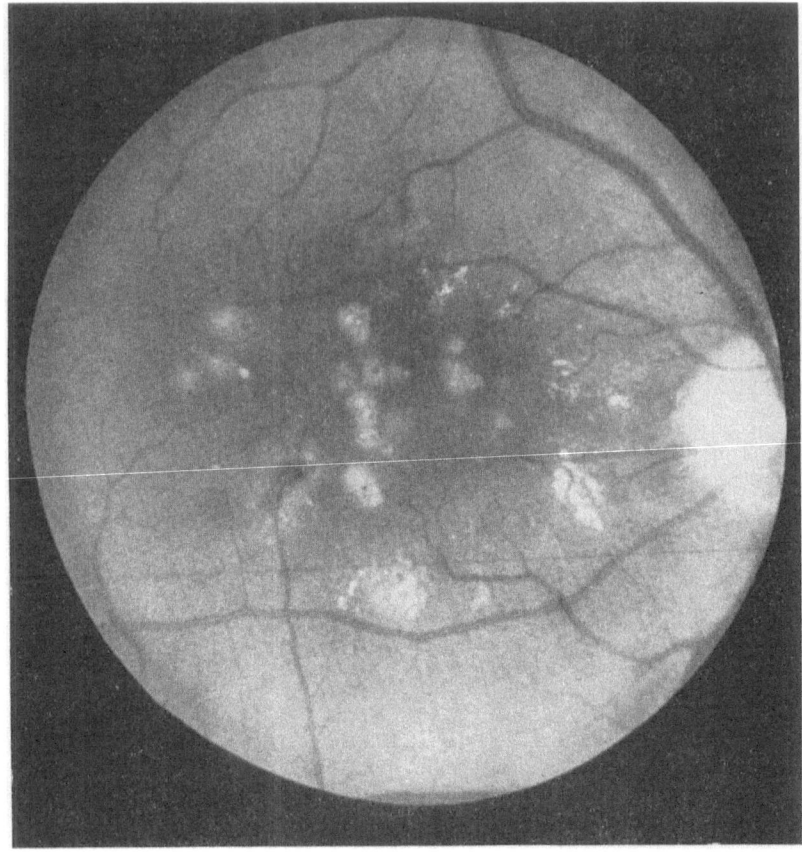

Fig. 3. Argon laser coagulation in Coats' disease. Coagulated aneurysms in the macular area.

trated light and the extremely small coagulation spot prevents the destruction of valuable macular tissue (Fig. 3).

One important differential diagnosis should be mentioned: retinal capillary angiomata. They show a very typical angiographic pattern. Most of the aneurysms are occluded by spontaneous thrombosis. There is no dye leakage and the surrounding capillaries do not show any disturbance. Retinal capillary angiomata do not progress and they show very little secondary changes. As a rule they do not use treatment with photocoagulation.

Complications

Complications very rarely occur except in the late stages where additional sub- or intraretinal exudation might be provoked. Superficial hemorrhages in the coagulated area are reabsorbed within 1 or 2 weeks.

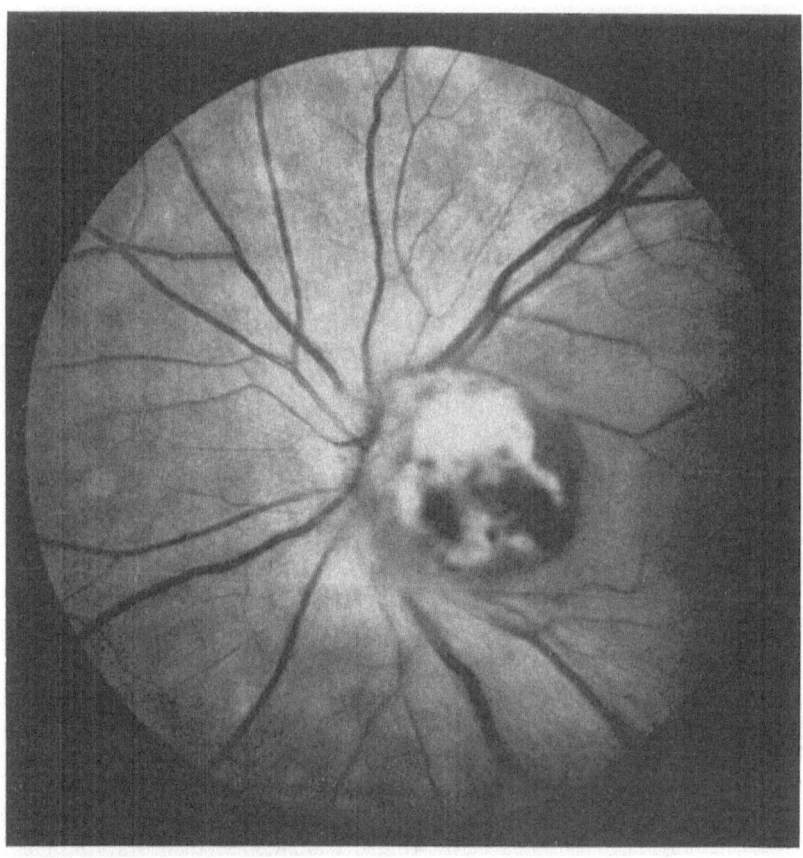

Fig. 4. Xenon arc coagulation in angiomatosis retinae.

Results

We have treated 26 cases of Coats' disease with peripheral lesions, five of these cases in combination with transscleral diathermy, 16 cases showed an improvement, 8 remained without further deterioration and in only two cases we found further progression. In five cases which were treated for macular lesions improvement of central visual accuity could be achieved.

III. ANGIOMATOSIS RETINAE

The success of photocoagulation treatment of angiomatosis retinae depends very much on the stage of the disease. Treatment is likely to succeed during the early stages. With the increase of size and number of angiomata the prospect of a cure will be worse and becomes minimal with the development of secondary changes such as detachment, vitreous hemorrhage and retinal degeneration.

The localisation of the tumours is of no less significance. A destroyed angioma at the disc or in the vicinity of the macula would leave behind more severe defects, than tumours in the peripheral region of the fundus.

Technique of treatment

One may distinguish four groups of tumours according to size and position.
1. Angiomas less than ½ disc diameter in size can be destroyed in one or two sessions without any risk of complications. One to three 'normal intensity coagulations' are sufficient. The size of the burns should be regulated by means of the image field diaphragm and should correspond to the size of the tumour.
2. In angiomas from ½ to 2 disc diameters in size the coagulations are directed to the centre of the tumour mass. The intensity of coagulations depends on the response obtained. Starting from a very low basic level it should be increased until a small contraction and change of color appears. Pale tumours containing a lot of glia, become reddish and hemorrhagic, where as the reddish tumours become paler as a result of blood vessel occlusion. Not more than five to six burns should be produced in order to avoid complications.

Four to eight weeks after the first coagulation the burned areas are transformed into scars, the amount of remaining tumour tissue can be seen, and a second coagulation can be carried out. The further treatment may be repeated at one to two months intervalls until the entire lesion is destroyed. 2–5 sessions are normaly required.
3. In angiomata over two disc diameters in size coagulations are performed in the same manner as in the previous groups. 8–10 sessions with 5–10 coagulation burns each are generally required for complete destruction of the tumour.

Occasionally large tumours form whitish exudates on their surface. This may interfere with further photocoagulation or even make it impossible. In those cases one has to return to trans- or intrascleral diathermy.

In the presence of changes such as retinal detachment due to traction or exudation, yellowish lipoidal deposits and retinal vascular proliferation, the prognosis must be guarded. In some cases of retinal detachment scleral infolding, cerclage operation or another buckling procedure is possible. However as a rule, in final stages of angiomatosis photocoagulation can produce no useful results.
4. The optic nerve head is one of the favorite sites of angiomas. It is necessary to destroy these angiomas in spite of the danger to central vision and visual field, since they may show rapid and extensive growth. The coagulation should be done with great care. The more accurate the dosage of light the smaller the scars produced and consequently the smaller the defects.

Complications

Regarding the complications, they were essentially of four types:

1. *Ablatio exsudativa fugax*

Coagulation of the larger angiomatous lesions is always followed by an exudative detachment. It usually starts just beneath the coagulated tumor and then spreads to involve more distant parts of the retina. It is at its maximum about ten to twenty hours after coagulation and disappears after a few days or weeks. The disappearance may be accelerated by giving cortison.

2. *Hemorrhages*

Small hemorrhages from the coagulated tumor appear regularly, either at the time of treatment or after a few hours or even days. These hemorrhages may obscure the tumor for a few weeks. Large irreversible vitreous hemorrhages are due to the coagulation and necrosis of large feeding vessels.

3. *Postcoagulative macular degeneration*

Macular puckering may occur in the same manner as known from other coagulation procedures and other diseases. The cause may be an anaphylactic reaction to the destroyed tissue of the tumor and of the retina.

4. *Vascular and fibrotic proliferation*

A rare complication is a proliferation of retinal vessels and of connective tissue from the coagulated areas. This applies to cases of large tumours and wide spread coagulations. There is no possibility to stop this process and usually the eyes are lost.

Results

From a total of 64 affected eyes 50 were treated by photocoagulation, whilst the remaining 14 were so badly affected at the time of the first examination that there was no question of treatment. 41 out of the 50 treated eyes (82%) were saved. But in 9 eyes (18%) it was impossible to halt the progressive growth of the angiomas. From the 41 eyes cured clinically the vision of 34 remained either unchanged or improved, whilst that of the remaining 7 decreased following complications. The 9 eyes not cured and the 7 eyes which showed decreased vision belonged to the group of large tumours and tumours at the disc.

SUMMARY

Photocoagulation treatment of Eales' disease, Coats' and Leber's disease and of angiomatosis retinae is discussed. Special indications for the use of the argon laser are pointed out.

REFERENCES

ASHTON, N.: Pathogenesis and aetiology of Eales' disease. Acta XIX Congr. Ophthal. II, pp. 828–840 (New Delhi 1962).

ELLIOT, A. J.: Recurrent intraocular hemorrhage in young adults (Eales' disease). *Trans. Amer. Ophthal. Soc.* 52: *811–875* (1954).

FRANCESCHETTI, A. & FORNI, S.: Le traitemant chirurgical des hémorraghies récidivantes rétino-vitréenne des jeunes sujets (maladie d'Eales). *Ophthalmologica* 127: *339–341* (1954).

MEYER-SCHWICKERATH, G.: Eales' disease, treatment with light coagulation. Acta XIX Congr. Ophthal. II, pp. 862–867 (New Delhi 1962).

— Lichtkoagulation. Bücherei des Augenarztes. 33. Beiheft Klin. Mbl. Augenheilk. Enke Verlag, Stuttgart (1959).

REESE, A. B.: Teleangiectasis of the retina and Coats' disease. *Amer. J. Ophthal.* 42: *1–8* (1956).

VERHOEFF, F. H.: Succesful diathermy treatment of recurring retinal hemorrhage and retinitis proliferans. *Arch. Ophthal.* 40: *239–244* (1948).

WEVE, H. J.: On diathermy in ophthalmic practice: The Bowman lecture. *Transact. Ophthal. Soc. U.K.* 59: *43–80* (1939).

WESSING, A.: 10 Jahre Lichtkoagulation bei Angiomatosis retinae. *Klin. Mbl. Augenheilk.* 150: *57–71* (1967).

ARGON LASER PHOTOCOAGULATION IN PERIPHERAL RETINAL NONVASCULAR DISEASES: RETINAL TEARS, RETINAL DEGENERATIONS' AND RETINOSCHISIS

HUNTER L. LITTLE. M.D.

(*Palo Alto, California*)

The purpose of this presentation is to discuss indications and techniques for argon laser photocoagulation in nonvascular peripheral retinal diseases. The absorption properties of retinal pigment epithelium for the argon laser wavelength make argon laser photocoagulation an excellent means to treat retinal tears, retinal degeneration, and retinoschisis. The indications for treatment of these disorders remain complex. Since GONIN first recognized that retinal detachments were caused by retinal tears (1920), the indications for prophylactic treatment of retinal tears has been questioned. MEYER-SCHWICKERATH introduced retinal photocoagulation in the form of xenon arc light making treatment more feasible than with the previously used electrocautery (1960). In spite of the even more sophisticated method of treatment with the slit lamp argon laser photocoagulator introduced in 1969 (LITTLE, ZWENG & PEABODY, 1970), the indications for treatment of certain nonvascular peripheral retinal pathology remains controversial.

With the introduction of binocular indirect ophthalmoscopy, scleral depression, and three mirror Goldmann contact lens with biomicroscopy, ophthalmologists frequently find asymptomatic retinal tears and areas of peripheral retinal degeneration that would have been overlooked. Asymptomatic tears found on routine examination pose the greatest debate in regard to prophylactic treatment. This controversy is quite obvious when one considers that 7.8% of eyes have been found to have retinal tears in a study by RUTNIN & SCHEPENS, 1967. Of further interest is the 6 to 7% incidence of lattice degeneration reported by STRAATSMA & ALLEN, 1962 and by BYER, 1965. These observations indicate the significance of performing a complete ophthalmological examination including the peripheral retina with the dilated pupil using the above methods. The question of which eyes should be prophylacticly treated remains debatable in many cases.

The three classic types of peripheral retinal degeneration are peripheral cystoid degeneration, cobblestone or peripheral chorioretinal degeneration, and lattice degeneration. Less well known is a benign peripheral pigmentary retinal degeneration in which there is an increased amount of retinal pigment seen scattered 360° in the equitorial region of the retina in many older patients. Increased retinal pigmentation is seen occasionally along the insertion of the

Palo Alto Medical Clinic, Palo Alto Medical Research Foundation and Stanford University School of Medicine, Palo Alto, California.

posterior vitreous base. A fifth syndrome is that of white without pressure which is presumed to be an indication of abnormal vitreal retinal adhesions; localized areas indicate a point of vitreal-retinal adhesion which is ominous, since such adhesions frequently lead to retinal tears. Generalized areas, called geographic white, are usually less troublesome.

Peripheral cystoid degeneration is the most common form of all retinal degenerations since it is found in almost all eyes over 20 and in increasing frequency with age. This type of degeneration is seen most frequently in the superior temporal quadrant immediately posterior to the ora serata. It is best seen with scleral depression at which time the degeneration appears white, hence the name 'white with pressure.' Histopathologicly peripheral cystoid degeneration represents an accumulation of mucoid material in the outer plexiform layer (HOGAN & ZIMMERMANN, 1962). As the cysts increase in size, they coalesce forming larger cysts which are separated by stretched Müller's fibers. Only when such cysts become extremely large are they termed retinoschisis. Peripheral cystoid degeneration is innocuous since it does not give rise to retinal tears or retinal detachment.

Cobblestone or peripheral chorioretinal degeneration is less frequent. It usually occurs after the age of 40 and increases in incidence with age. The lesions are seen in the inferior temporal fundus immediately posterior to the ora serata. They appear as white atrophic chorioretinal scars somewhat similar to an old inactive toxoplasmic retinal choroiditic scar. The overlying vitreous is clear. Microscopically such areas of degeneration show an abrupt disappearance of the retinal pigment epithelium, of the rod and cone layer, and of the outer nuclear layer (HOGAN & ZIMMERMANN, 1962). There is an absence of the choriocapillaris and hyalinization of the choroidal stroma. Such areas of degeneration do not give rise to tears or retinal detachment.

The most significant of the retinal degenerations is that of lattice degeneration since it frequently is associated with horseshoe retinal tears and since it is a predisposing factor to retinal detachment. Lattice degeneration characteristically is situated in the equitorial region of the retina. It can be present in any quadrant of the globe situated along the posterior vitreous base. It is characterized by white branching lattice-like patterns having an eliptical shape with a width approximately 2 mm and a length ranging from 1 to 4 hours of the clock. When studied with indirect ophthalmoscopy and scleral depression, lattice degeneration has questionable round holes. Such holes seldom lead to detachment. The retinal detachments associated with lattice degeneration most frequently result in horseshoe tears developing around the margins. Microscopically lattice degeneration is an extremely thin and degenerated retina with occluded retinal vessels (HOGAN & ZIMMERMANN, 1962). The inner retinal layers are absent; the outer plexiform, outer nuclear, and rod and cone layers are intact. Localized areas of vitreous liquification overlie the areas of lattice degeneration. Vitreous is adherent along the margins of the lattice. A combination of the degeneration and of the vitreous traction produces retinal horseshoe tears.

Prophylactic photocoagulation of lattice degeneration is debatable. Since the incidence of lattice degeneration is between 6 to 7% (2, 10) and since the incidence of retinal detachment ranges from .005% (1) to .01% (8) lattice degeneration only seldom leads to retinal detachment. Probably the best recommendation in the management of lattice degeneration is to make an accurate retinal drawing and to follow such patients on a 6 month basis for repeated observation of the fundus. In the event that the patient should have either a horseshoe retinal tear or a retinal detachment in the same or in the other eye, prophylactic argon laser photocoagulation is indicated. Sometimes prophylactic treatment is used in aphakic eyes or in eyes before cataract surgery.

There are five major indications for prophylactic argon laser photocoagulation of retinal tears (ZWENG, LITTLE & PEABODY 1969):

1. Association of hemorrhage with the retinal tear.
2. Association of vitreous traction on the tear.
3. Association of subretinal fluid around the margins of the tear.
4. Presence of symptoms as represented by vitreous opacities and peripheral light flashes.
5. History of retinal detachment in the other eye.

If any one of these major indications is present, the patient is best managed by prophylactic photocoagulation.

In addition to the above five major indications for prophylactic photocoagulation, the following five minor indications for treatment are listed (ZWENG, LITTLE & PEABODY 1969):

1. Location of the hole above the horizontal meridian.
2. Presence of myopia above 4 diopters.
3. Absence of pigment in and about the hole since presence of pigment represents longer duration of the lesion.
4. High degree of physical activity in the patient's work or recreation.
5. History of retinal detachment in the patient's family.

Probably the best management of the minor indications is to make a retinal drawing and follow the case. If three to five of the minor indications are present, one might consider treating such a tear prophylactically.

The method in which prophylactic argon laser photocoagulation is carried out has been described under the section of instrumentation. The three-mirror Goldmann contact lens is used with the tear being treated under direct observation of the slit lamp photocoagulator. The points of coagulation are applied to the attached healthy retina surrounding the retinal tear. The usual settings for treatment of medium to large size tears are in the range of 200 milliwatt power for a 200 micron spot at .05 to .1 second or a 400 milliwatt power for a 500 micron spot size at .1 second. A double ring of contiguous coagulation points is applied around the tear (Fig. 1, 2). Exposure times of longer than .2 second are discouraged since one is likely to produce adverse heating of the ocular media. If there is a large horseshoe retinal tear with considerable evidence of vitreous traction, a third or fourth ring of coagulation about the tear would be indicated. The 1000 micron spot at 800 to 1000 milliwatts of power at 0.1 second creates larger points of adhesions. Such would be the base if one were placing a barricade around a giant retinal tear or dialysis.

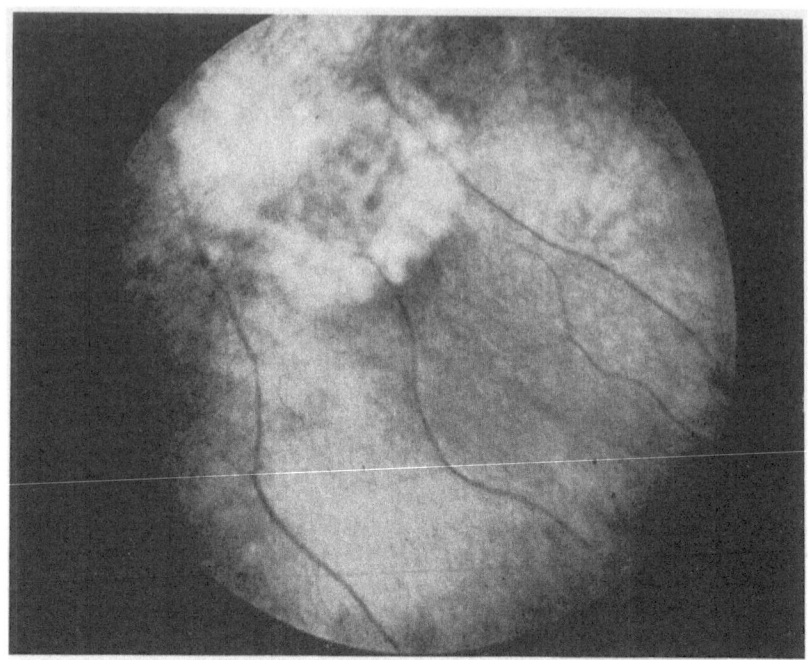

Fig. 1. Retinal tear immediately after argon laser photocoagulation.

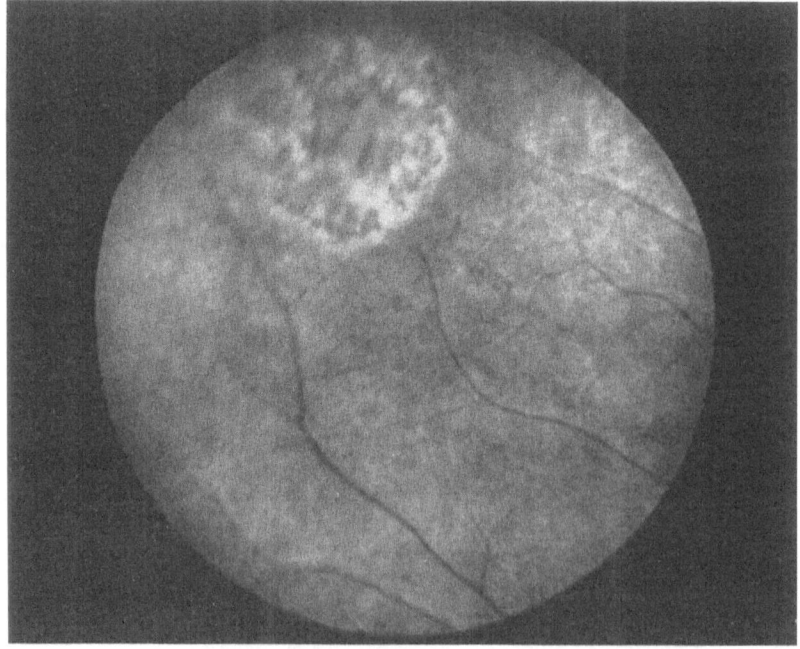

Fig. 2. Pigmentary scar surrounding retinal tear one week after argon laser photocoagulation.

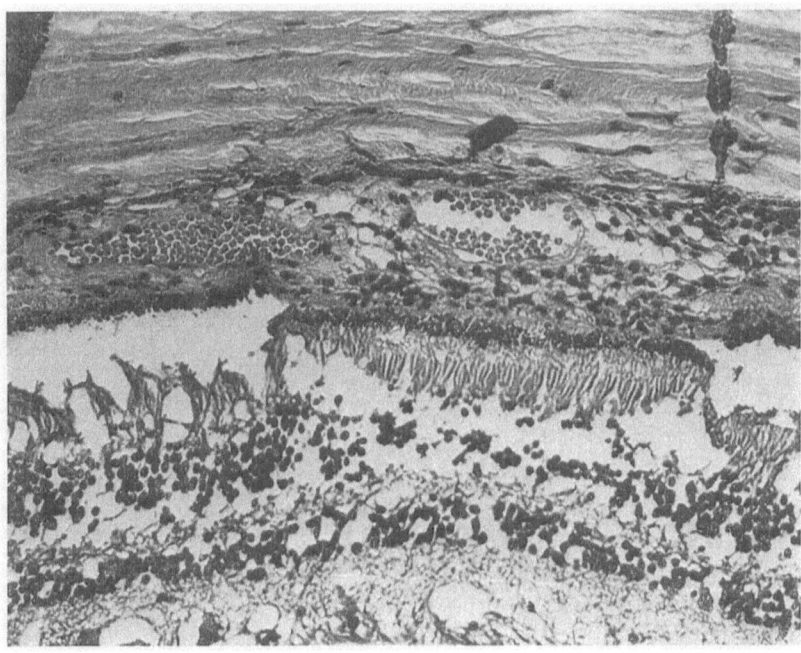

Fig. 3. Histopathology of argon laser photocoagulation lesion in human retina 72 hours after photocoagulation.

The histopathology of argon laser photocoagulation in the human retina shows adhesion to the retinal pigment epithelium within 72 hours (Fig. 3). One week after producing a nonintensive lesion there is proliferation of the retinal pigment epithelial cells and loss of outer sensory retinal elements (Fig. 4, 5).

Senile retinoschisis is an exaggerated form of peripheral cystoid degeneration with giant cystic separations within the retinal layers usually arising in the outer plexiform layer. These giant areas of retinoschisis are frequently situated in the inferior temporal quadrant and are usually bilateral. Most cases of retinoschisis do not require treatment since they progress very slowly. The usual management is accurate retinal drawings and observation every four months. If there is progression of the retinoschisis or if the macula is threatened, argon laser photocoagulation is indicated. The author recommends the technique described by OKUN & CIBIS, 1964. This involves the coagulation of the entire bed of the retinoschisis using multiple applications with the setting at .1 second, 500 to 1000 milliwatts, and 500 to 1000 micron spot size respectively (Fig. 6). Within four to eight weeks the schisis flattens in most cases (Fig. 7). Furthermore, if there is space between the posterior margin of the schisis of the macula, a barrier of coagulation is placed along the posterior margin of the schisis.

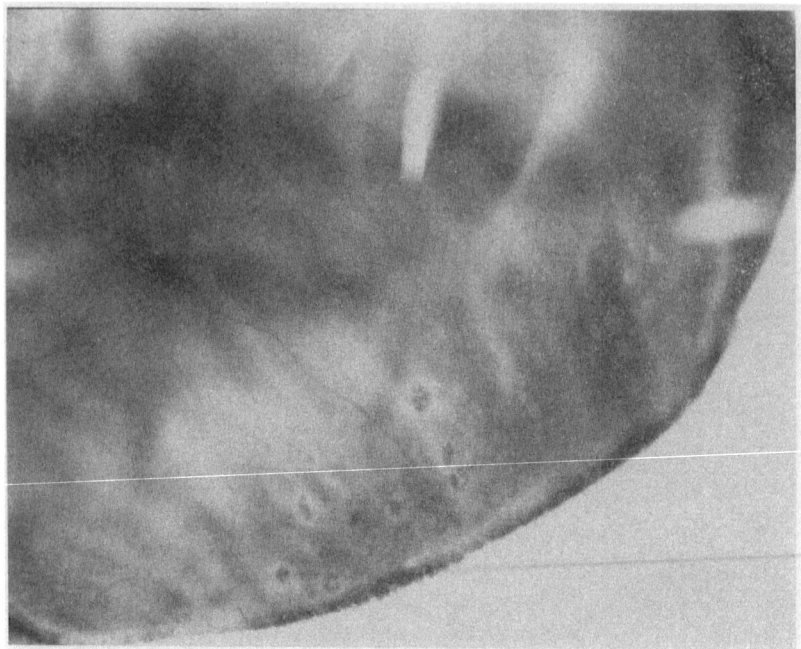

Fig. 4. Gross pathology of argon laser photocoagulation lesions seen one week after coagulation. Note hyperplasia or retinal pigment epithelium.

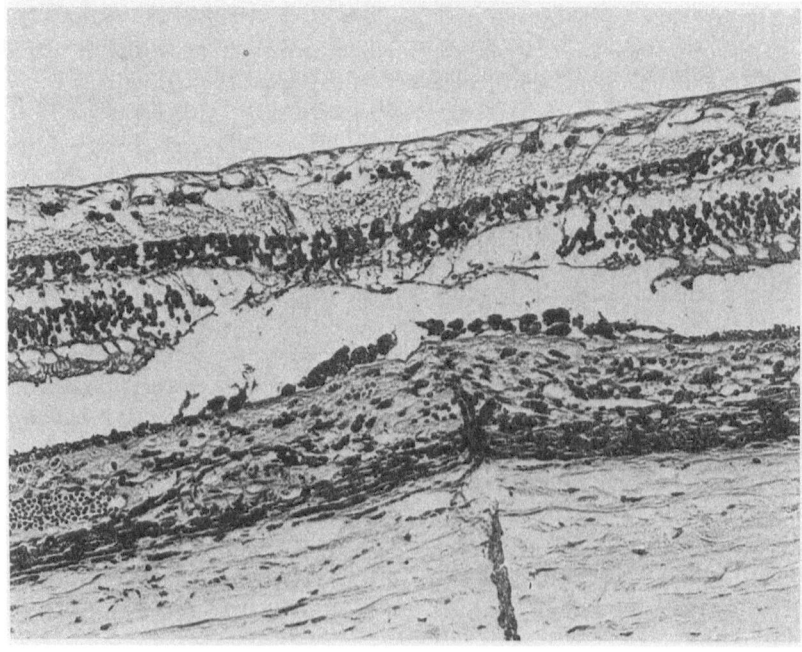

Fig. 5. Histopathology of argon laser photocoagulation lesion in human retina one week after photocoagulation with 500 micron, .1 second, and 500 milliwatts.

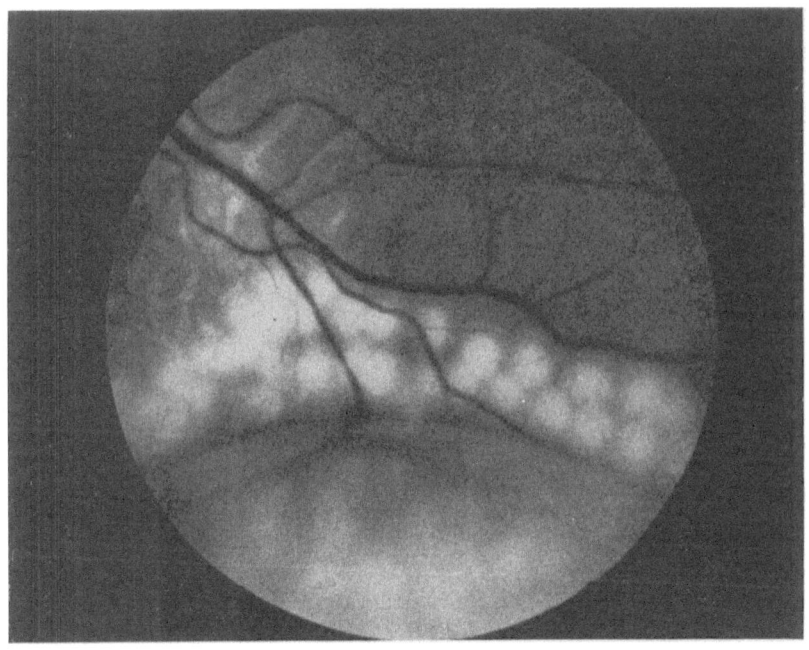

Fig. 6. Retinoschisis immediately after argon laser photocoagulation.

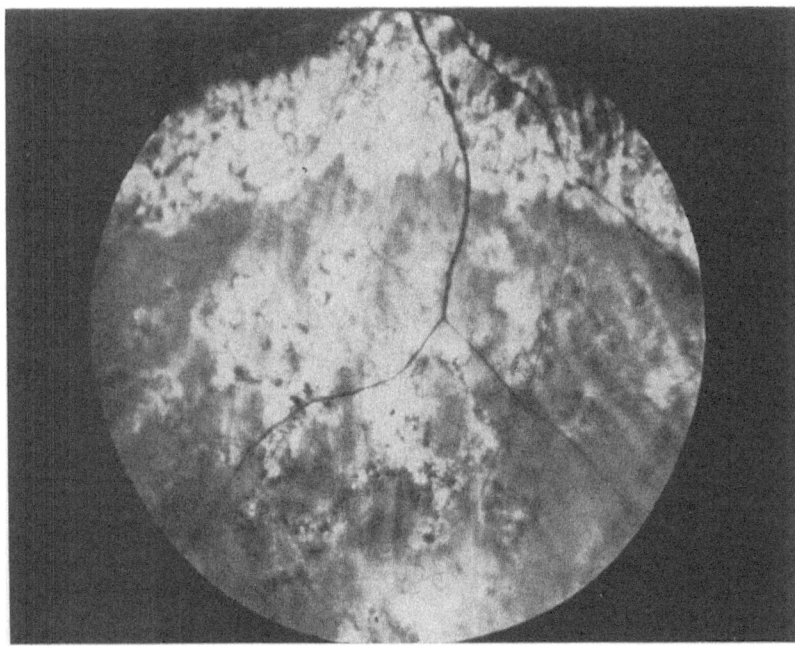

Fig. 7. Flattened retinoschisis three months after argon laser photocoagulation.

No complications have resulted from argon laser photocoagulation of retinal tears and retinoschisis. This treatment has been used since May, 1969. Preretinal membrane contracting has occurred only in the management of proliferative retinopathies. This information does not preclude the possibility that preretinal membrane contracting or hemorrhage could occur with argon laser photocoagulation of nonvascular peripheral retinal disease.

REFERENCES

BOHRINGER, H. R.: Statistisches zur Häufigkeit und Risiko der Netzhautablösung. *Ophthalmologica* 131: *331*, (Apr.–May 1956).

BYER, N. E.: Clinical study of lattice degeneration of the retina. *Trans. Amer. Acad. Ophthal. Otolaryng.* 69: *1066* (Nov.–Dec. 1965).

GONIN, J.: *Bull. Soc. Franç. Ophtal.* 33: *1* (1920).

HOGAN, M. J. & ZIMMERMAN, L. E.: An Atlas and Textbook of Ophthalmic Pathology. W. B. Saunders Co. 2, Philadelphia (1962).

LITTLE, H. L., ZWENG, H. C. & PEABODY, R. R.: Argon laser slitlamp retinal photocoagulation. *Trans. Amer. Acad. Ophthal. Otolaryng.* 74: *85–97* (1970).

MEYER-SCHWICKERATH, G.: Light Coagulation. St. Louis. The C. V. Mosby Co. (1960).

OKUN, E. & CIBIS, P. A.: The role of photocoagulation in the management of retinoschisis. *Arch. Ophthal.* 72: *309* (Sept. 1964).

RINTELEN, F.: Zur Frage der Haufigkeit der Netzhautablösung und zum Phänomen kompensatorisch-gerontogischer Prozesse. *Ophthalmologica* 143: *291* (1962).

RUTNIN, U. & SCHEPENS, C. L.: Fundus appearance of normal eyes. IV. Retinal breaks and other findings. *Amer. J. Ophthal.* 64: *1063* (July–Dec. 1967).

STRAATSMA, B. R. & ALLEN, R. A.: Lattice degeneration of the retina. *Trans. Amer. Acad. Ophthal. Otolaryng.* 66: *600* (Sept.–Oct. 1962).

ZWENG, H. C., LITTLE, H. L. & PEABODY, R. R.: Laser Photocoagulation and Retinal Angiography. St. Louis, C. V. Mosby Co. (1969).

Key Words:

Argon laser retinal photocoagulation
Nonvascular peripheral retinal disease
Retinal tears
Retinal degeneration
Retinoschisis
Indications
Prophylactic treatment

NATURAL HISTORY AND PREOPERATIVE
EVALUATION OF DIABETIC RETINOPATHY

J. FRANÇOIS & J. J. DE LAEY

(Ghent)

Before discussing the technique and the results of photocoagulation in diabetic retinopathy, it is important to consider its natural history, its prognosis and its preoperative evaluation.

I. NATURAL HISTORY

There are two main types of diabetic retinopathy:

1. A non-proliferative, simple or background retinopathy.
2. A proliferative retinopathy.

The first sign of the retinopathy is a venous congestion. It is not specific and of questionable value, as the calibre of the retinal veins is variable.

The most typical sign in the beginning stage is the appearance of micro-aneurysms and dot-like haemorrhages. This sign is probably preceded by alterations of the capillary bed and by small areas of capillary closure, which can only be detected by fluoro-angiography.

The altered capillary wall produces an accumulation of plasma into the retinal tissue. The fluid is reabsorbed and consequently a selective accumulation of lipids occurs (MAUMENEE, 1968). But according to WOLTER (1961) and TOUS-SAINT (1968) the cause of the lipid deposits is a neuronal degeneration. In any case these deposits indicate a local ischaemia, which, if long standing, will produce a permanent neuronal damage.

The lipid deposits are either small and isolated or large and confluent or even circinate (Fig. 1).

As almost one third of the pathological capillaries are situated just lateral to the macula (DOBREE, 1970), it is not surprising that the macular oedema and the lipid deposits or exudates are at the basis of the visual impairment in the non-proliferative stage of the disease.

Macular oedema is, indeed, much more frequent than it was thought. It is, however, often seen only by fluoro-angiography. When the macular oedema is important, multiple cysts may be seen, which sometimes coalesce and give the aspect of a lamellar hole of the macula.

Even when there is no arterial hypertension, cotton-wool exudates and flame-

From the Ophthalmological Clinic of the University of Ghent. Director: Prof. J. FRANÇOIS.

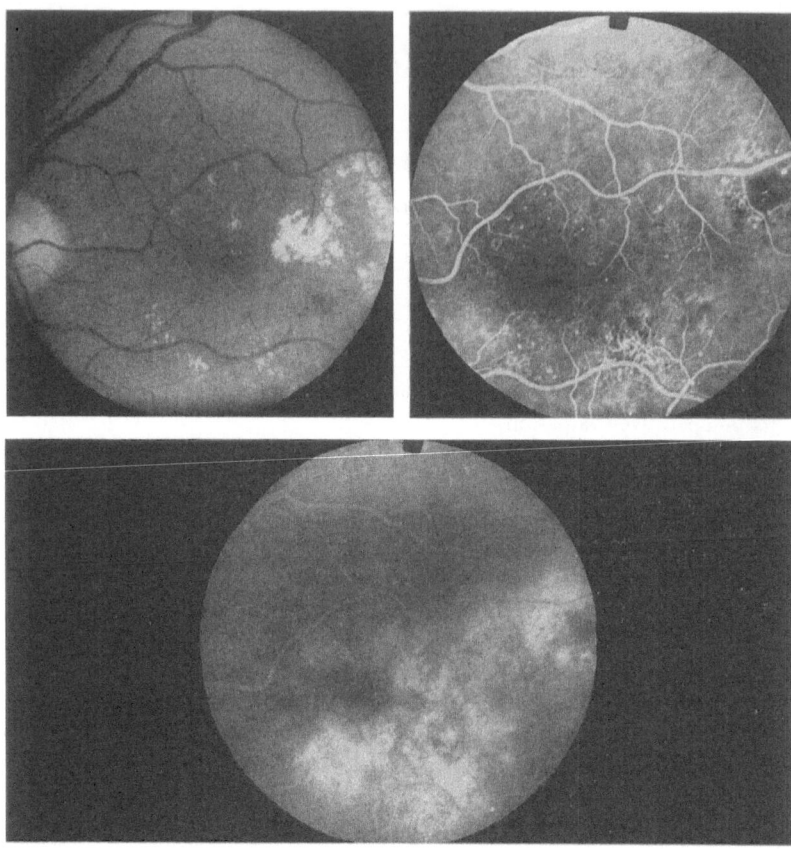

Fig. 1. Non-proliferative retinopathy with macular exudates and oedema.

shaped haemorrhages may be found (DAVIS, 1968; KOHNER, 1971). Cotton-wool exudates probably represent acute localized closure of the capillary bed.

In more severe retinopathy changes are seen not only in the capillaries, but also in the venules and arterioles (Fig. 2). Alteration in the permeability of the larger vessels and arterio-venous communications may be visualized angiographically. Segmentary dilatations, venous loop-formations and thread-like arterioles are often observed.

A further response to ischaemia is the newvessel formation (Fig. 3). In nearly 75% of the cases with proliferative diabetic retinopathy the vessels appear in the vicinity of the optic disc (TAYLOR & DOBREE, 1970), but they may also develop around the large retinal veins, more frequently around the superior temporal vein. There is a high degree of correlation between the site of the new vessel formation and the nearest arterio-venous crossing (TAYLOR & DOBREE, 1970). Sometimes the new vessels are found in close connection with areas, where there is no perfusion and sometimes in areas with relatively normal

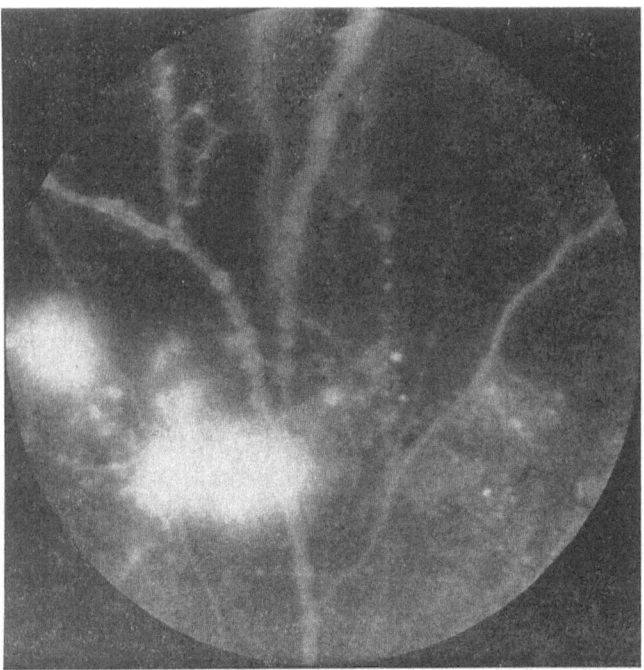

Fig. 2.   Early proliferative retinopathy with segmentary venous dilatations and large areas of capillary closure.

capillaries, as vessel perfusion not necessarily means adequate tissue nutrition (KOHNER, 1971).

The evolution of the new-formed vessels can be divided in 3 stages (DOBREE, 1964): (1) growth, (2) fibrosis (Fig. 4) and (3) obliteration of the vessels, retraction of the fibrous tissue and detachment of the vitreous. These three stages may be observed in the same fundus.

DAVIS (1967) stressed the important role of the vitreous in proliferative diabetic retinopathy. The vitreous detachment is probably related to a marked exudation from the new formed vessels. It is possible that these do not grow into the vitreous, but are rather pulled forward by the retracting vitreous. Traction of the vitreous on pathological vessels or on the retina may cause vitreous haemorrhages, retinoschisis and retinal detachment. Recurrent haemorrhages may coïncide with each increase of the vitreous detachment. When this is complete, the haemorrhages usually diminish, as does the new vessel formation.

The evolution is, however, not always so dramatic and the vitreous may lift whole fans of new-formed vessels without changing its shape or producing haemorrhages (OKUN et al., 1971).

The proliferative diabetic retinopathy generally runs a course of about 5

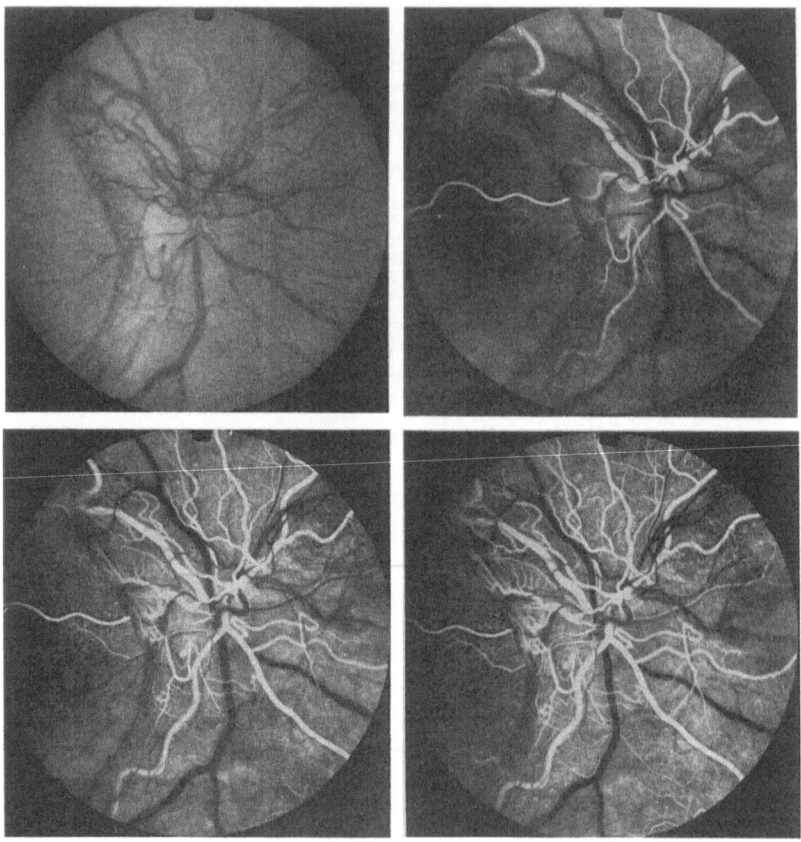

Fig. 3. Proliferative retinopathy. Indication of the feeder vessels.

years before blindness occurs (DUKE-ELDER, 1967). Blindness is mainly due to retinal detachment (44%), persistent vitreous haemorrhage with organization (35%), macular oedema or exudates (15%), glaucoma with rubeosis iridis or occlusion of the central retinal vessels (OKUN et al., 1971).

The evolution, which we have described, is classical. Many cases run another course. DOBREE (1964), DAVIS (1968), BEETHAM (1963), IRVINE & NORTON (1971) have observed a spontaneous regression of the proliferative diabetic retinopathy. BEETHAM (1963) saw it in about 10% of his cases with long follow-up. MADSEN (1971) found a status quo of the proliferative changes in 30% of his cases. Although the regression is mostly incomplete, all the vessels may occasionally disappear (DAVIS, 1967). This fact makes the evaluation of any treatment very difficult.

Some local conditions may influence the evolution of diabetic retinopathy. In 8 out of 10 patients with an asymmetric retinopathy, GAY & ROSENBAUM (1966) observed a significant difference between the diastolic pressure of both

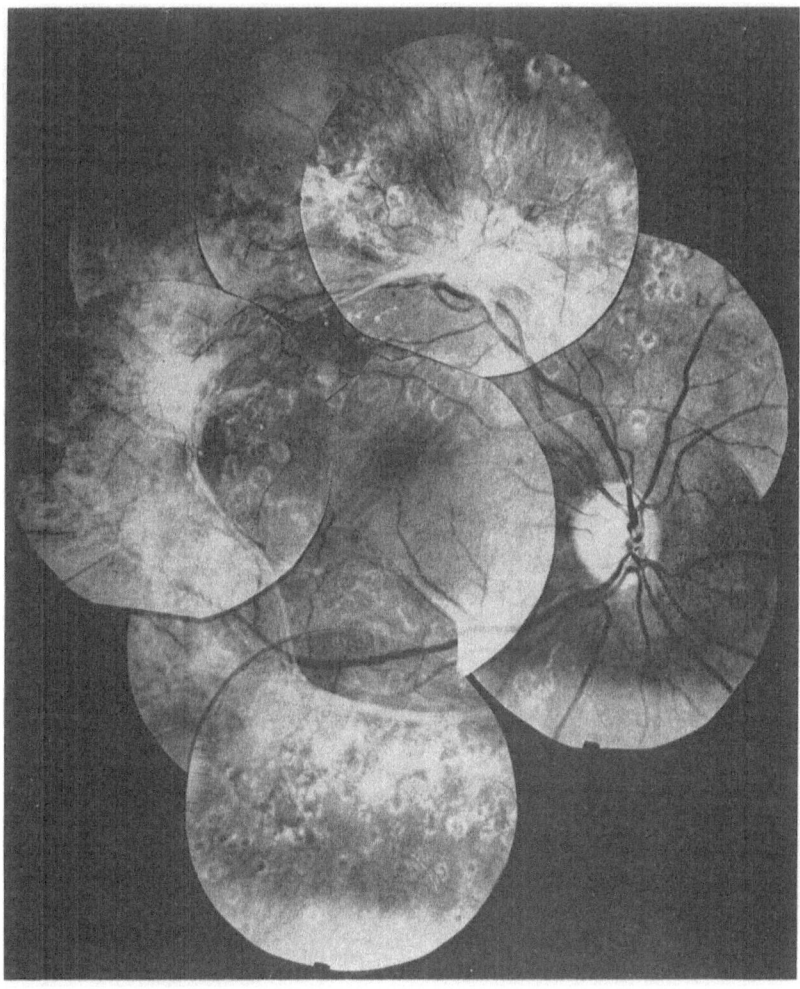

Fig. 4. Proliferative retinopathy with marked fibrosis and macular tractions folds.

retinal arteries, revealing a carotid stenosis at the side of the less severe retino-pathy. Glaucoma (MOONEY, 1963), optic atrophy (OKUN & CIBIS, 1966), myopic choroidosis and chorioretinal scars (AMALRIC, 1967) seem also to have a bene-ficial influence. These facts can be explained by a vascular atrophy. KOHNER (1971) could demonstrate an important reduction of the retinal flow after photocoagulation, what can also be seen fluoro-angiographically.

According to CAIRD & GARRETT (1963), when the vision is initially good (20/20–20/60), 51,5 % of the patients with non proliferative diabetic retinopathy keep still a good vision after 5 years, 34 % have an impaired vision (20/80–20/200) and 14,5 % become blind (less than 20/200). When the vision is initially poor (20/80–20/200), 50 % become blind within 5 years.

In proliferative diabetic retinopathy 35–50 % of the patients retain a good vision for a rather long period (BEETHAM, 1963; DAVIS, 1967). BEETHAM (1963) distinguishes 4 stages: early, moderate, marked and extreme. The average rate of progression from one to another stage is 1,5 year. The proliferative diabetic retinopathy takes thus more or less 5 years to progress from stage I to stage IV.

The visual prognosis depends mainly on the extent and the localisation of the proliferative changes. When these are peripheral 50 % of the eyes become blind within 5 to 6 years, whereas in case of pre- or peripapillary proliferation 50 % become blind within 2 to 3 years (DECKERT et al., 1967). If one eye becomes blind, the chance for the other eye to become blind within the next 12 months is about 60 % (PATZ & BERKOW, 1968).

According to a survey of juvenile diabetics insured by the Metropolitan Life Insurance Company, these patients have a mortality rate 2 to 6 times higher than the average population (POLLACK et al., 1967). The mortality rate is still higher for blind diabetics, the survival after the onset of the blindness being about 5,8 years (BERKOW et al., 1965). ROOT et al. (1959) obtained analogous figures.

Summarizing we may say:

1. In cases of non-proliferative diabetic retinopathy visual impairment is mainly due to macular exudates and oedema. The therapy should aim to prevent their appearance or to hasten their resorption. In cases of long standing exudates definite neuronal disturbances nevertheless occur, so that the visual loss becomes permanent. In this case the disappearance of the exudates will give a much more normal fundus, but will be of little benefit for the patient.

2. The vital and visual prognosis of proliferative diabetic retinopathy is poor. The therapy, which should try to maintain a useful vision for the few years these patients have to live, must destroy the proliferating vessels and prevent haemorrhages as well as retinal detachment.

3. As the spontaneous evolution of the diabetic retinopathy is unpredictable, one should not be too enthusiastic after some single good results. The therapy can only be judged on large series of well documented observations.

III. PREOPERATIVE EXAMINATION

1. A biomicroscopic examination of the anterior segment may reveal a rubeosis iridis, corneal opacities or a cataract. When the lens- or cornea opacities are too pronounced, photocoagulation may be difficult and also dangerous, as

higher intensities are needed, so that cornea or lens lesions may appear. These opacities are the main contra-indication for the treatment of non proliferative diabetic retinopathy.

2. The visual acuity is not a good parameter. A patient who has 10/10 vision, but shows marked retinal proliferations becomes, indeed, much sooner blind than a patient, who has only 3/10 vision, due to macular exudates, but shows otherwise a mild retinopathy.

3. Concerning the visual fields, it is sometimes surprising to hear how little the patients complain of scotomas after extensive photocoagulation for diabetic retinopathy. This is not astonishing, when one studies the visual fields of diabetics before the treatment. In about 50 % of the diabetic patients without visible retinopathy ROTH (1969) found, indeed, scotomas of the central visual field. This may be related to the findings of OOSTERHUIS & LAMMENS (1967), who found in these patients angiographically localized alterations of the capillary network.

In fact, in the posterior pole KOHNER (1971) found a close relationship between the areas of altered capillaries and the visual field defects studied with the Roth-Keeler scotometer. In more peripheral lesions this relationship is not so obvious. This might be due to distorsions during the photography or to the fact that the function of the affected area has partially been taken over by the normal adjacent areas. In non proliferative diabetic retinopathy WISZNIA et al. (1971) found an arcuate type of field defect with partial narrowing of the central isopters. According to these authors the arcuate scotoma may depend on the radial peripapillary capillaries. In proliferative diabetic retinopathy the peripheral field defects are due to peripheral retinal proliferations and haemorrhages (Fig. 5), whereas the arcuate scotomas are due to proliferations starting from or around the optic disc. In the case of macular haemorrhages or exudates a central scotoma will of course be present.

4. The electro-retinogram and the electro-oculogram are not of primary importance in diabetic retinopathy. One of the first electrophysiological signs is the disappearance of the oscillatory potentials (YONEMURA et al., 1962), but these may also be absent in normal cases. An increase of the amplitude of the b-wave during the glucose tolerance test may also be seen (HENKES et al., 1960; VAN POPPEL & BUTLER, 1964) and is probably due to a generalized retinal ischaemia.

When the diabetic retinopathy is accompanied by a severe arterial hypertension or important retinal proliferations the base value of the electro-oculogram may become too low (FRANÇOIS et al., 1957). HENKES & HOUTSMULLER (1965) found an abnormal EOG depending on the stage and the duration of the retinopathy.

5. The biomicroscopical examination of the fundus will show the severity of the vitreous alterations and reveal the macular oedema.

6. Normal and stereo-photography of the fundus is of the greatest importance for the follow-up of the retinopathy and the evaluation of the therapeutic results. A good panoramic view of the fundus can be obtained with 5 to 7 pictures of the posterior pole (DAVIS et al., 1968; OKUN et al., 1971). The new

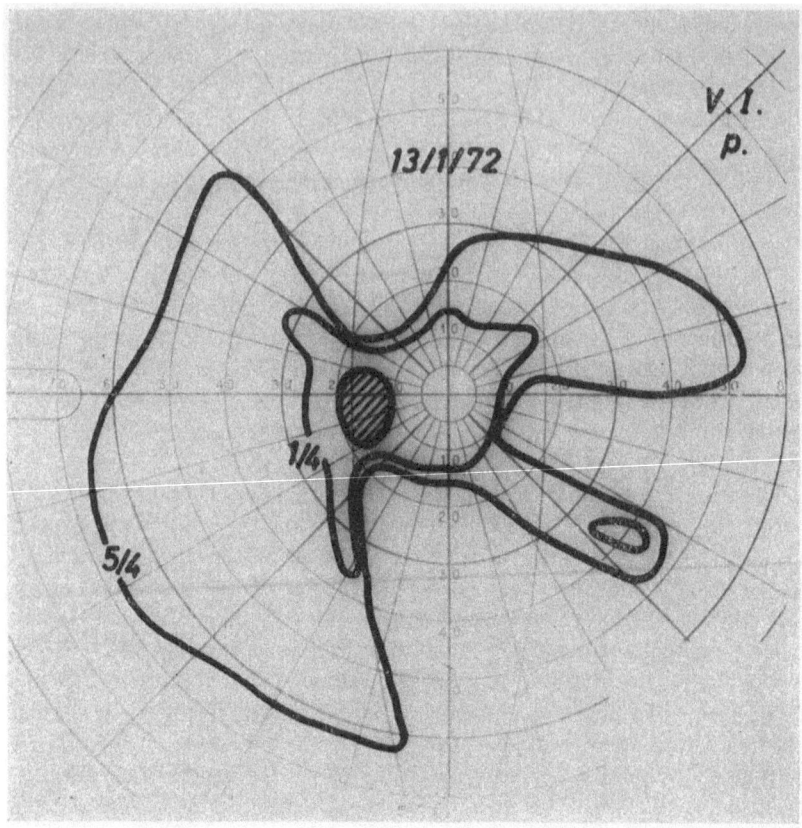

Fig. 5. Visual field in a case of proliferative diabetic retinopathy.

wide angle camera with an angle of 45° instead of 30° may also be of great help (Fig. 6). It has, however, the disadvantage to produce a marked distorsion at the periphery, especially when photographs have to be taken outside the posterior pole.

7. Fluorescein angiography has, of course, a capital importance for a more detailed follow-up. But it is also of great help in the preoperative study of the fundus. Indeed:

a. It visualizes the areas of non-perfusion, which eventually should be destroyed.

b. It demonstrates the macular oedema, which can only be guessed by ophthalmoscopy.

c. It better visualizes early proliferations and areas of dye diffusion.

d. It indicates the feeder vessels, especially in pre- or peripapillary proliferations.

In cases of pronounced proliferative diabetic retinopathy the intense dye

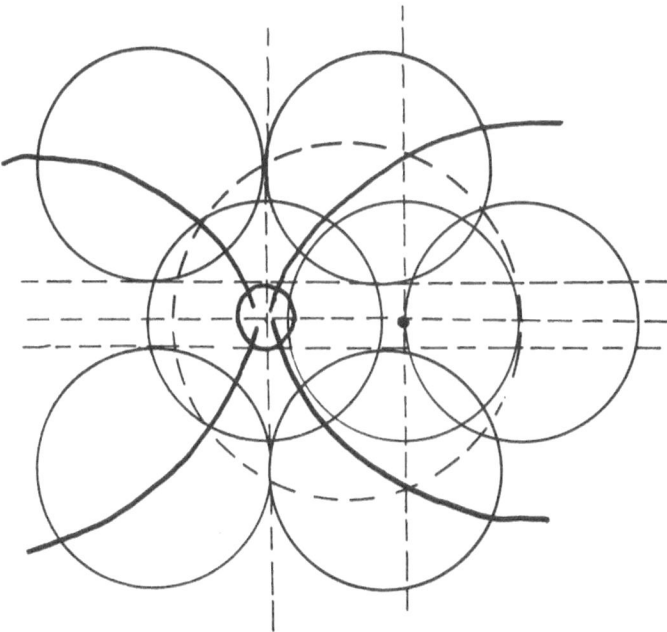

Fig. 6. Photographic fundus survey according to OKUN et al. (1971). The dotted line represents the field of the wide-angle camera (45°).

diffusion makes argon laser photocoagulation difficult. Therefore, we prefer to wait at least 24 hours before treatment.

REFERENCES

AMALRIC, P.: Nouvelles considérations concernant l'évolution et le traitement de la rétino-pathie diabétique. *Ophthalmologica* (*Basel*) 154: *151–160* (1967).

BEETHAM, W. P.: Visual prognosis of proliferating diabetic retinopathy. *Brit. J. Ophthal.* 47: *611–619* (1963).

BERKOW, J. W., SHUGARMAN, R. G., MAUMENEE, A. E. & PATZ, A.: A retrospective study of blind diabetic patients. *J. Amer. Med. Ass.* 193: *867–870* (1965).

CAIRD, F. & GARRETT, C. J.: Prognosis for vision in diabetic retinopathy. *Diabetes* 12: *398* (1963).

DAVIS, M. D.: Natural course of diabetic retinopathy. In Kimura and Caygill: Vascular complications of diabetes mellitus. C. V. Mosby, St. Louis, 139–167 (1967).

DAVIS, M. D.: The natural course of diabetic retinopathy. *Trans. Amer. Acad. Ophthal.* 72: *237–240* (1968).

DAVIS, M. D., NORTON, E. W. D. & MYERS, F. L.: Classification of diabetic retinopathy. In Goldberg M. F. and Fine S. L.: Symposium on the treatment of diabetic retinopathy. U.S. Department of Health, Education and Welfare, Arlington, 7–22 (1968).

DECKERT, T., SIMONSEN, S. & POULSEN, J.: Prognosis of proliferative retinopathy in juvenile diabetics. *Diabetes* 16: *728–733* (1967).

DOBREE, J. H.: Proliferative diabetic retinopathy. *Brit. J. Ophthal.* 48: *637–649* (1964).

DOBREE, J. H.: Simple diabetic retinopathy. *Brit. J. Ophthal.* 54: *1–10* (1970).

DUKE-ELDER, S. & DOBREE, J. H.: System of Ophthalmology. Vol. X. Diseases of the retina. Ed. Henry Kimpton, London, 408–448 (1967).

FRANÇOIS, J., VERRIEST, G. & DEROUCK, A.: L'électro-oculographie en tant qu'examen fonctionnel de la rétine. *Adv. Ophthal., Karger, Basel* 7: *1–67* (1957).

GAY, A. J. & ROSENBAUM, A. L.: Retinal artery pressure in asymmetric diabetic retinopathy. *Arch. Ophthal. (Chicago)* 75: *758–762* (1966).

HENKES, H. E. & HOUTSMULLER, A. J.: Fundus diabeticus. *Amer. J. Ophthal.* 60: *662–670* (1965).

HENKES, H. E., VAN BALEN, A. T. M. & HOUTSMULLER, A. J.: Über die objektive Beurteilung der retinalen Funktion bei den diabetischen Retinopathie. *Ber. Dtsch. Ophthal. Ges. Berlin* 63: *75–80* (1960).

IRVINE, A. R. & NORTON, E. W. D.: Photocoagulation for diabetic retinopathy. *Amer. J. Ophthal.* 71: *437–445* (1971).

KOHNER, E.: The effect of diabetes on retino-vascular functions. In Lundbaek K. and Keen H. (ed.), Blood vessel disease in diabetes mellitus. Ed. Il Ponte, Milan, 135–178 (1971).

MADSEN, P. H.: Prognosis for vision and fundus changes in patients with proliferative diabetic retinopathy. *Brit. J. Ophthal.* 55: *372–382* (1971).

MAUMENEE, A. E.: Fluorescein angiography in the diagnosis and treatment of lesions of the ocular fundus. *Trans. Ophthal. Soc. U.K.* 88: *529–556* (1968).

MOONEY, A. J.: Diabetic retinopathy. A challenge. *Brit. J. Ophthal.* 47: *513–520* (1963).

OKUN, E. & CIBIS, P. A.: The role of photocoagulation in the therapy of proliferative diabetic retinopathy. *Arch. Ophthal. (Chicago)* 75: *337–352* (1966).

OKUN, E., JOHNSTON, G. P. & BONIUK, I.: Management of diabetic retinopathy. A stereoscopic presentation. Ed. C. V. Mosby, St. Louis, 1–48 (1971).

OOSTERHUIS, J. A. & LAMMENS, A. J. J.: Fluorescein photography of the ocular fundus. *Ophthalmologica, (Basel)* 149: *210–220* (1965).

PATZ, A. & BERKOW, J. W.: Visual and systemic prognosis in diabetic retinopathy. *Trans. Amer. Acad. Ophthal.* 72: *253–258* (1968).

POLLACK, A. A., MC GURL, T. J. & MC INTYRE, N.: Diabetes mellitus: a review of mortality experience. *Arch. Int. Med.* 119: *161–163* (1967).

ROTH, J. A.: Central visual field in diabetes. *Brit. J. Ophthal.* 53: *16–25* (1969).

ROOT, H. F., MIRSKY, S. & DITZEL, J.: Proliferative retinopathy in diabetes mellitus. *J. Amer. Med. Ass.* 169: *903–909* (1959).

TAYLOR, E. & DOBREE, J. H.: Proliferative diabetic retinopathy. Site and size of initial lesions. *Brit. J. Ophthal.* 54: *11–19* (1970).

TOUSSAINT, D.: Contribution à l'étude anatomique et clinique de la rétinopathie diabétique chez l'homme et chez l'animal. Presses Académiques Européennes, Brussels (1968).

VAN POPPEL, A. L. A. & BUTLER, I.: The use of flicker-electroretinography in the judgment of the retinal metabolic condition in diabetes mellitus. *Documenta Ophthalmologica* 18: *404–411* (1964).

WISZNIA, K. I., LIEBERMAN, T. W. & LEOPOLD, I. H.: Visual fields in diabetic retinopathy. *Brit. J. Ophthal.* 55: *183–188* (1971).

WOLTER, J. R.: Diabetic retinopathy. *Amer. J. Ophthal.* 51: *1123–1139* (1961).

YONEMURA, D., AOKI, T. & TSUZUKI, K. Electroretinogram in diabetic retinopathy. *Arch. Ophthal. (Chicago)* 68: *19–24* (1962).

XENON ARC THERAPY OF
DIABETIC RETINOPATHY

A. WESSING & M. VOGEL

(*Essen*)

Photocoagulation with the Zeiss xenon arc coagulator in diabetic retinopathy is now performed for more than 15 years. The purpose of this paper is to give a summary of the results, we have obtained with this technique and to outline method and indication for photocoagulation treatment according to our own point of view.

GENERAL RESULTS

Let us first take a look at some fundamental results of photocoagulation in diabetic retinopathy.

1. Microaneurysms, dilated capillaries and proliferated vessels in the plane of the retina obliterate and disappear after photocoagulation.

2. The vascular lesions are also reduced if they have not been coagulated directly. Obviously photocoagulation has a certain effect on the whole retina and leads to a normalisation of circulation even if the lesions are far away from the coagulation effect. That this process includes large areas of the whole capillary bed is shown by fluorescein angiograms. An obviously regular although relatively coarse vascular pattern develops out of the bizarre pre-treatment aspect of microaneurysms, dilated capillaries, exudates, edema and hemorrhages. During this reorganisation a partial or complete restitution of the blood-tissue-barrier is accomplished.

3. The volume and the tortuosity of the veins are reduced. This also reflects the effect of photocoagulation on the total retinal circulation.

4. Hard exudates diminish in most cases. Depending on the duration of their development and presence in the retina they either leave behind a functioning retina or scars.

5. The regression of the lesions takes place much faster in the juvenile diabetic than in patients over 50 years of age. It very often takes several months until the endstage of improvement is reached.

6. Photocoagulation can prevent the development of vascular proliferations into the vitreous.

7. If intravitreal proliferations are present photocoagulation becomes difficult.

In our experience proliferations can only be treated successfully in the early stages. In cases of advanced proliferations photocoagulation will, as a rule, be too late.

Complications are rare in non-proliferative retinopathy and consist in occasional, small preretinal hemorrhages in the area of the coagulation. Such hemorrhages are usually absorbed in the course of 1–2 weeks. If large retinal vessels are avoided massive hemorrhage may very rarely occur.

In those cases where diabetic retinopathy is combined with hypertensive retinopathy or sclerosis complications may be seen in the form of post-coagulative, intraretinal exudation in the macular area. The diminution of function will only gradually or never subside.

An exudative, post-coagulative retinal detachment (ablatio exsudativa fugax) is usually harmless and will disappear within 1 week without any loss of function. It is surprising that post-coagulative macular puckering is rarely seen in diabetic retinopathy ($< 1 \%$).

The danger of complications increases immediately in proliferative retinopathy. These complications are massive vitreous hemorrhage, retinal detachment due to traction, optic atrophy and secondary glaucoma.

It is remarkable that post-coagulative visual field defects are scarcely realized by the patient. The defects are minute even if several hundred coagulations are applied. It seem as if the reason for this are plaque- like ischemic areas in the retina. They develop already in the early stages of the disease by obliteration of capillaries and they are the cause of minute slowly growing scotomas. Most of the vascular changes which are to be coagulated are located at the borderline of such ischemic areas. Therefore the pre-existing scotoma is only slightly enlarged by the coagulation.

MODE OF ACTION OF PHOTOCOAGULATION

The way how photocoagulation acts is up to now unknown. In our own view which is mainly based on the works of ASHTON the important point is not the coagulation of the altered vessels but the destruction of retinal tissue. The latter leads to a decrease of metabolic activity and reduction of oxygen demand of the whole retina. The obviously specific change of the whole capillary network after photocoagulation as it becomes visible in the fluorescein-angiogram would be the morphologic counterpart for the adaption of metabolism and hemodynamic on a new yet lower level. The reconstruction of the blood-tissue barrier emphasizes that this is a true process of restitution. The observation that diabetic changes in eyes with large chorio-retinal scars of the fundus in high myopia or after diathermy operations take a less violent course than in the unaffected partner eye seems to confirm our view. The view of RUBINSTEIN is quite similar. He recommends to coagulate smaller clinical ischemic areas because a local insufficiency of the blood supply may produce a vasoactive factor stimulating proliferation of vessels.

WETZIG believes that dynamic circulation factors are more important. The interruption of numerous capillary connections means a diminution in the blood flow on the venous side of the retinal vascular tree. The chronic congestion of the large veins is thereby interrupted.

Both theories are of course important for the explanation of the effect of photocoagulation but there are certainly additional, unknown factors involved. This applies particulary to the function of the chorio-capillaris and the retinal pigment epithelium.

PEYMAN, SPITZNAS & STRAATSMA recently demonstrated by electronmicroscopy that the barrier of permeability of the retinal pigment epithelium is broken down by photocoagulation and a new orientation of the metabolic exchange takes place.

INDICATIONS

From the knowledge of the natural, chronic course of diabetic retinopathy, the results of photocoagulation and the impression of its mode of action the following outlines for the indication of photocoagulation and its practical use may be elaborated.

The indication for photocoagulation is dictated by the progression of diabetic retinopathy. Those cases where only a few microaneurysms are seen remain under photographic control. Photographs are taken every 3–6 months and only where an obvious progression is observed treatment is started. Particularly in juvenile diabetics controls are definitely required because the malignant, proliferative form can develop in the course of a few weeks.

Photocoagulation is immediately performed in cases with numerous micro-aneurysms, severe retinal edema, exudates and hemorrhages. If large deposits of lipoidal material are present in the macular area photocoagulation is also immediately performed. The same holds true for new formed vessels which are about to proliferate into the vitreous. Because of the danger of macular damage cases with severe hypertension or sclerosis are coagulated either very carefully or not at all.

The same reluctance is recommended in cases of advanced vascular pro-liferations. If the new formed sea-fan shaped vessels are elevated more than 4–5 dptr. and have a width of more than 2–3 disc diameters they should not be coagulated. This is also recommended for proliferations in the area of the disc. These rules apply at least to the xenon coagulator. Fibrotic lesions should not be coagulated because of additional shrinkage.

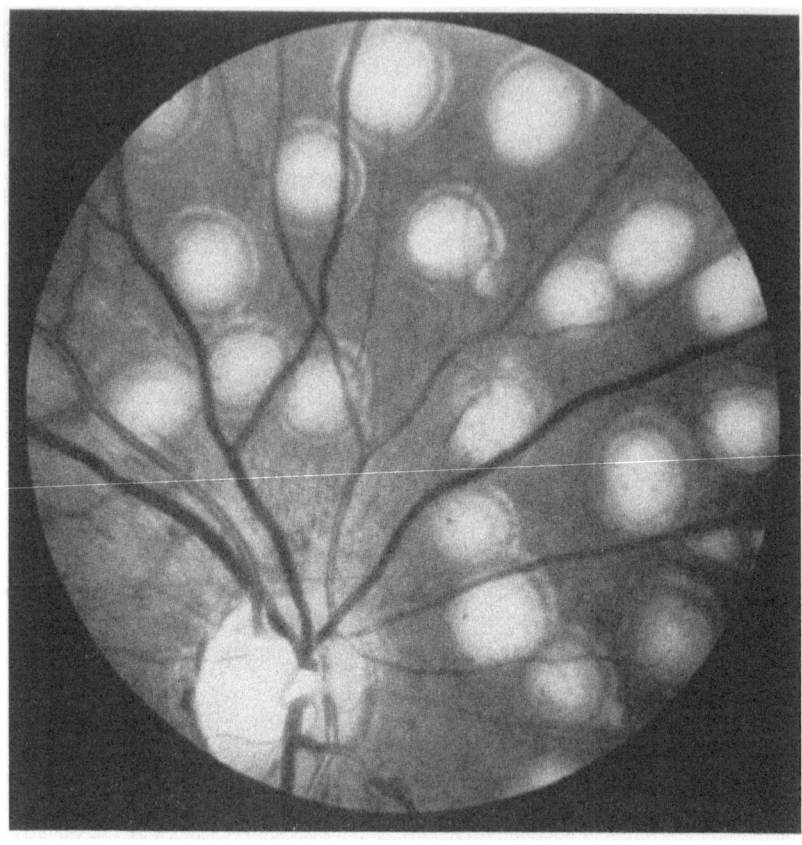

Fig. 1. Xenon arc photocoagulation in diabetic background retinopathy.

METHOD

One of the primary goals of photocoagulation is the occlusion of sources of hemorrhages and on this scale to prevent recurring, intraretinal hemorrhages. The photocoagulations are therefore aimed at microaneurysms, small hemorrhages, and new formed vessels. If our conclusion is correct that the long-term effect of photocoagulation is based mainly on the destruction of retinal tissue then it will not alone be important to coagulate the vascular lesions but also an adequate part of the retina (Fig. 1). For that reason 150–200 coagulations are distributed over the central fundus and the mid periphery. A bridge of intact retina remains between each coagulation. By these means large and particularly the fan-shaped visual fielddefects can be avoided. The diameter of each coagulation is usually 3°. In an emmetropic eye this means about 1 mm. The intensity is chosen such that during ½–1 second an obvious whitish discoloration of the retina will develop. A minimal distance of 1½–2 disc diameters is mandatory when coagulating around the macula and the disc. Coagulations within the papillo-macular bundle do not necessarily mean a hasard to visual acuity. By using a small diaphragm and low intensity the nerve fiber layer remains undamaged.

Only were few microaneurysms are located close to the macula causing heavy exudation and deposition of lipoidal material within the macula these microaneurysms should be coagulated. Circular lipoidal deposits with one or more centrally located microaneurysms lend themselves particulary for this procedure. The coagulation is performed either with diaphragm 1 or 1,5°.

Large lipoidal plaques in the macular area in exudative retinopathies are not coagulated but only distinct microaneurysms in their immediate vicinity. The majority of photocoagulation is placed in the peripheral fundus.

The only exception from the rule of distributing coagulations over larger parts of the fundus are intra- or preretinal vascular proliferations. If one tries at all to destroy vessels in such a case intensive coagulations have to be applied regardless of visual field defects.

As mentioned before the results in large far extended preretinal proliferations are rather poor. In the majority of such cases one will have to consider the intrascleral diathermy coagulation (WESSING & BÖCKENHOFF).

During the post-coagulative treatment – as in all photocoagulations – local atropin ointment is administered over a period of 8–14 days combined with local steroids.

CONCLUSION

There is, of course, no doubt that photocoagulation in diabetic retinopathy is a purely symptomatic and destructive treatment. We feel, however, as long as there are no other methods, which are more effective and less radical for the whole organism one should not hesitate to apply photocoagulation early and on a large scale.

SUMMARY

The principles of photocoagulation in diabetic retinopathy are discussed, and guidelines for techniques and indications are recommended.

REFERENCES

MEYER-SCHWICKERATH, G. & SCHOTT, K.: Diabetic retinopathy and photocoagulation. *Amer. J. Ophthal.* 66: *597—603* (1968).
PEYMAN, G. A., SPITZNAS, M. & STRAATSMA, B. R.: Peroxidase diffusion in the normal and photocoagulated retina. *Invest. Ophthal.* 10: *181—189* (1971).
— Chorioretinal diffusion of peroxidase before and after photocoagulation. *Invest. Ophthal.* 10: *489—495* (1971).

RUBINSTEIN, K. & MYSKA, V.: Focal retinal ischemia. *Trans. Ophthal. Soc. U.K.* 91: *355—367* (1971).

WESSING, A.: Die Behandlung der diabetischen Retinopathie mit Lichtkoagulation. In: PFEIFFER, E. F. 'Handbuch des Diabetes mellitus' J. F. Bergmann Verlag Vol. 2 pp. 1290—1301 München (1971).

WESSING, A. & BÖCKENHOFF, I: Die Behandlung der Retinopathia diabetica proliferans mit Diathermiekoagulation. *Klin. Mbl. Augenheilk.* 158: *212—220* (1971).

WETZIG, P. C. & JEPSON, C. N.: A review of 232 patients including 401 eyes with diabetic retinopathy treated by light-coagulation. In: GOLDBERG, M. F. & ST. L. FINE: 'Treatment of diabetic retinopathy'. *US Public health service publication* 1890: *593—601* (1969).

ARGON LASER THERAPY OF
DIABETIC RETINOPATHY

HUNTER L. LITTLE, M.D.

(*Palo Alto*)

Diabetes mellitus is the second leading cause of new adult blindness in the United States; retinopathy accounts for 84% of blindness in diabetics. Over 60% of diabetics develop retinopathy after having had diabetes for 15 or 20 years (GOLDBERG & FINE, 1968). These data indicate the significance of diabetic retinopathy. Proliferative retinopathy is responsible for blindness in over 90% of the blind diabetics under 40 (WHITTINGTON, 1964). Exudative retinopathy accounts for most blindness in the elder diabetics.

Proliferative retinopathy off the optic disc is one of the major causes of recurrent vitreous hemorrhage and blindness in diabetics. Xenon arc and ruby laser photocoagulation have been unsuccessful in satisfactorily eliminating this problem. Because of its absorption properties by hemoglobin, the argon laser provides the best available means to erradicate proliferative vessels off the optic disc (LITTLE, ZWENG & PEABODY, 1970).

A very practical classification of diabetic retinopathy suggested by ZWENG, LITTLE & PEABODY, 1972 is presented:

I. Nonproliferative
   a. localized leak without macular edema
   b. localized leak with macular edema
   c. diffuse leaks
II. Proliferative retinopathy within the plane of the retina.
III. Proliferative retinopathy of the optic disc or into the vitreous.
IV. Proliferative retinopathy of the optic disc or into the vitreous plus significant fibrous element.

The limitation of this classification is its failure to include hemorrhages and degrees of vitreous traction. However, it has proven useful in categorizing cases for treatment and for follow-up studies.

The following table illustrates the overall results of diabetic retinopathy treated by H. C. ZWENG and the author with argon laser photocoagulation in cases followed from six months to three years. Such data is less meaningful than that obtained from studies of groups with specific stages of diabetic retinopathy.

Argon laser photocoagulation of nonproliferative diabetic retinopathy is less hazardous than that of proliferative retinopathy. Fluorescein angiography

Palo Alto Medical Clinic, Palo Alto Medical Research Foundation and Stanford University School of Medicine, Palo Alto, California.

Diabetic Retinopathy Treated With Argon Laser Photocoagulation.
(6 month to 3 year follow-up)

Total eyes	345
Improved	63%
Unchanged	12%
Worse	25%

usually shows the accumulation of the dye within the center of areas of circinate exudative retinopathy suggesting that vessels within the center of the circinate ring are responsible for the surrounding of the accumulation of exudates. The treatment consists of coagulating the center of the circinate rings with a 200 micron spot size with power levels from 200 to 400 milliwatts at .1 to .2 sec. The coagulation point should be moderately heavy to produce adequate thrombosis of the leaking vessels. Once the macular area shows advanced cystoid changes, the prognosis for ultimate visual improvement is unlikely. Patients having localized areas of circinate exudative retinopathy respond well to this form of treatment. However, in cases with diffuse retinal edema involving the entire posterior pole with massive retinal effusion demonstrated on fluorescein angiography, the prognosis is poor.

Brief comment will be made concerning complications of argon laser photocoagulation. In argon laser photocoagulation of proliferative diabetic retinopathy, the two most significant complications are hemorrhage and recurrent growth of vessels (LITTLE & ZWENG, 1971). Because of these, alterations in the technique of argon laser photocoagulation have been made to give better results.

Because of the high absorption properties of the argon laser beam by blood, one can occlude retinal vessels at the time of coagulation. Such vascular occlusions produce immediate changes in the hemodynamics of retinal circulation. Sudden closure of venous or efferent channels cause vascular engourgement and hemorrhage. Thus, differentiation of arterial or afferent vessels from venous or efferent vessels is essential in reducing the complication of hemorrhage.

In proliferative retinopathies, the afferent and efferent vessels are difficult to differentiate because the usual color differential between arteries and veins may be absent, the vessels are intertwined among themselves, and the surrounding connective tissue prevents direct viewing of the vessels. Fluorescein angiography provides a means by which one can identify frequently the afferent vessels to neovascular fronds. The importance of high resolution and high magnification fluorescein angiograms in argon laser treatment of proliferative retinopathy cannot be overstressed. Stereo photographs of fluorescein studies facilitate the identification of the afferent vessels. Coagulation of the afferent vessels before treating the entire frond of neovascularization reduces the number of significant hemorrhages.

The afferent or feeder vessel treatment usually employs the following settings: a 50 micron spot size, .1 to .2 second exposure, and 100 to 200 milliwatts of power. Multiple applications increasing the power until attenuation and obliteration are achieved are applied to the feeder vessels. Then the entire frond is treated obliterating all vessels excepting very large efferent vessels. The frond is usually treated with the 100 to 200 micron spot with 100 to 200 milliwatts power at .1 and .2 sec.

To state that retinopathy has been improved or that it is better following photocoagulation is not significantly meaningful. A proliferative frond can be partially obliterated and therefore improved in appearance yet still be a potential source of a massive vitreous hemorrhage. Therefore, the ultimate goal in argon laser photocoagulation in diabetic retinopathy should be to erradicate all neovascular fronds and background retinopathy. Such an achievement is not always possible, but one should strive to eliminate all remaining fronds in which an identifiable blood column is seen. The end result shows obliteration of vascular fronds and absence of venous engorgement, background hemorrhages, exudates, and edema. Then the retinopathy is classified quiescent.

Fig. 1, 2 and 3 illustrate the pre- and post-treatment fluorescein angiograms of a large proliferative frond. Similar times in the angiographic studies are used for comparison. The treatment consisted of obliterating the feeder vessels. Subsequent obliteration during the same treatment session of the entire vascular frond is necessary to prevent recanalization of the feeder vessels.

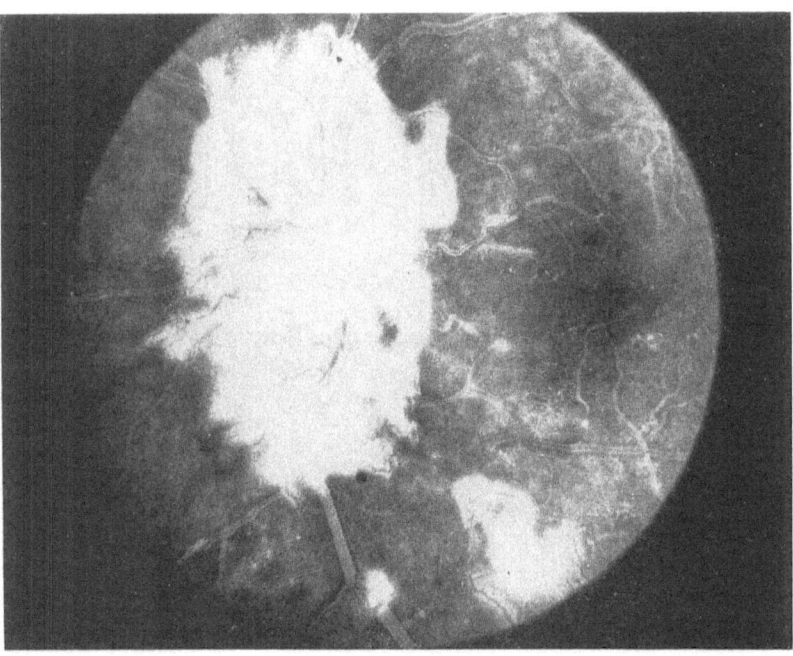

Fig. 1. Venous phase of pretreatment fluorescein angiogram in proliferative diabetic retinopathy.

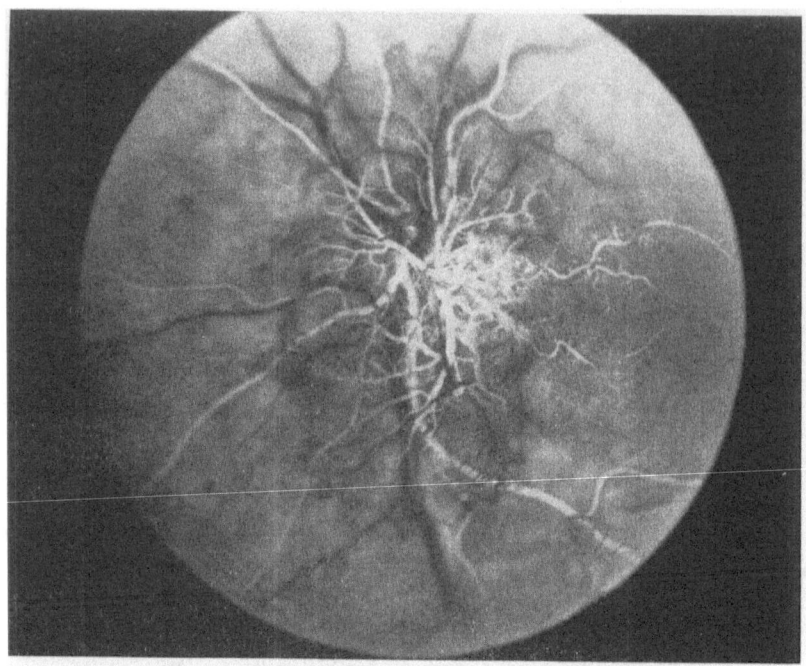

Fig. 2. Arterial phase of pretreatment fluorescein angiogram showing feeder vessels to neovascular frond in same eye as Fig. 1.

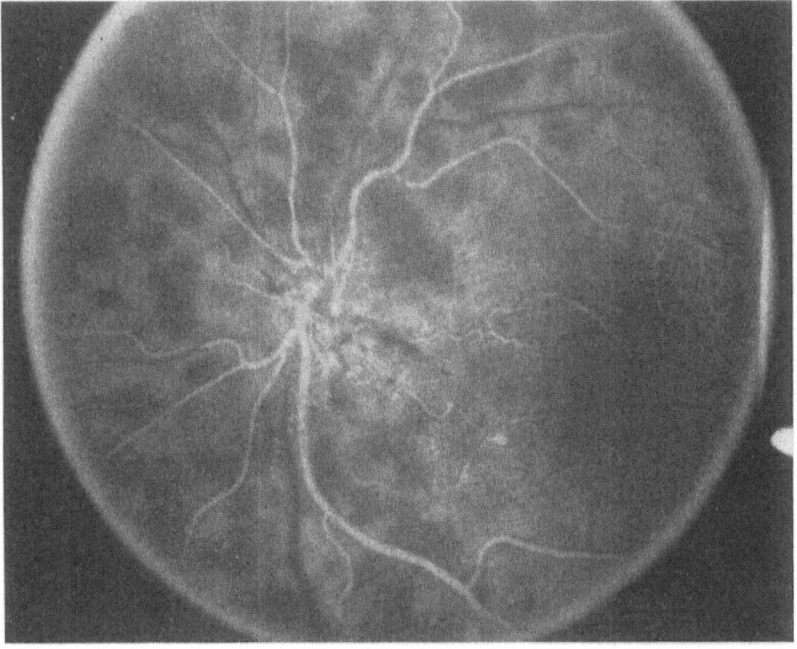

Fig. 3. Arterial phase of angiogram done one day after argon laser photocoagulation to feeder vessels and frond. Same eye as Fig. 1 and 2.

Weeks to months after obliteration of the neovascular fronds, recurrent growth of vessels commonly occurs. The recurrent vessels may be more pronounced than the original frond. By combining the retinal ablation approach to photocoagulation as described by WESSING & MEYER-SCHWICKERATH, 1968 and by AIELLO & BEETHAM, 1968, one reduces the problem of recurrent neovascularization.

The usual settings for the ablation lesions are as follows: 500 micron spot size, 0.1 sec., and 400 to 500 milliwatts power or 1000 micron spot size, 0.1 sec. and 800 to 1200 milliwatts. Lesions are systematically placed from the paramacular region to the equator. Large retinal vessels are avoided to prevent arterial and venous occlusions. Approximately 1000 to 1500 lesions are applied in addition to those required to obliterate disc and other proliferative neovascularization. Therefore, it is not unusual to apply approximately 2000 lesions before completing treatment. Fig. 3, 4 and 5 illustrate the pre- and post-treatment appearance. The combined approach utilizing feeder-vesselfrond and multiple 360° retinal ablation was done.

The following table summarizes results of eyes treated with nonfeeder vessel technique, with feeder vessel frond technique, and with feeder vessel frond combined with 360° peripheral ablation coagulation:

Proliferative Diabetic Retinopathy.
4–12 mo. follow-up

	Nonfeeder	Feeder	Feeder Plus 360
No. eyes	50	28	41
Better	60%	79%	88%
Same	12%	–	–
Worse	22%	13%	13%
Quiescent	12%	7%	55%
Hemorrhage	16%	6%	5%

The prognosis of achieving a good result with argon laser photocoagulation is largely dependent upon the selection of the patients to be treated. Cases in which the ocular media is extremely cloudy due to vitreous hemorrhage should be eliminated from consideration for treatment. Cases in which there is massive fibrous element to the proliferative retinopathy are extremely poor subjects since the argon laser cannot be focused upon the vessels because of the intervening connective elements.

The most favorable cases of proliferative retinopathy are those in which the proliferative retinopathy is in the plane of the retina or in which the proliferative retinopathy is coming off the optic disc or off the surface of the retina but having little fibrous component to the retinopathy. With the feeder vessel technique such fronds usually can be eliminated, and with the 360° peripheral-retinal-ablation coagulation, recurrent neovascularization can be minimized. Since the prognosis is much worse in far advanced retinopathy, an educational

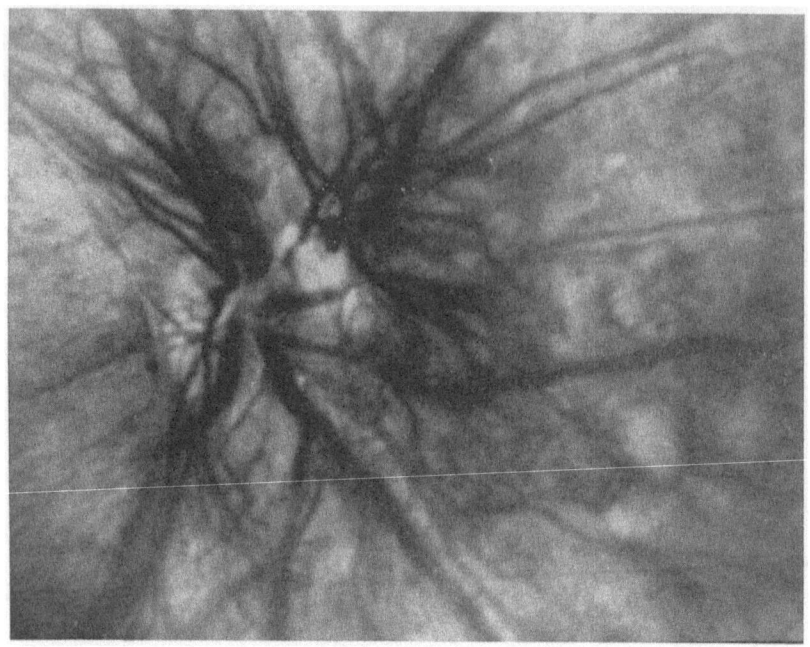

Fig. 4. Funduscopic appearance of proliferative diabetic retinopathy before argon laser photocoagulation.

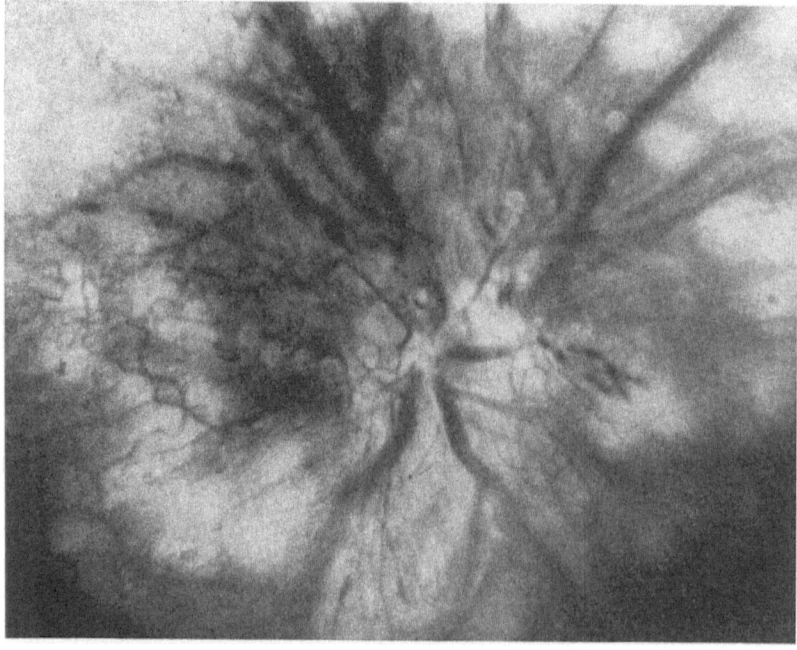

Fig. 5. Segmentation of vessels one day after argon laser photocoagulation to frond depicted in Fig. 4.

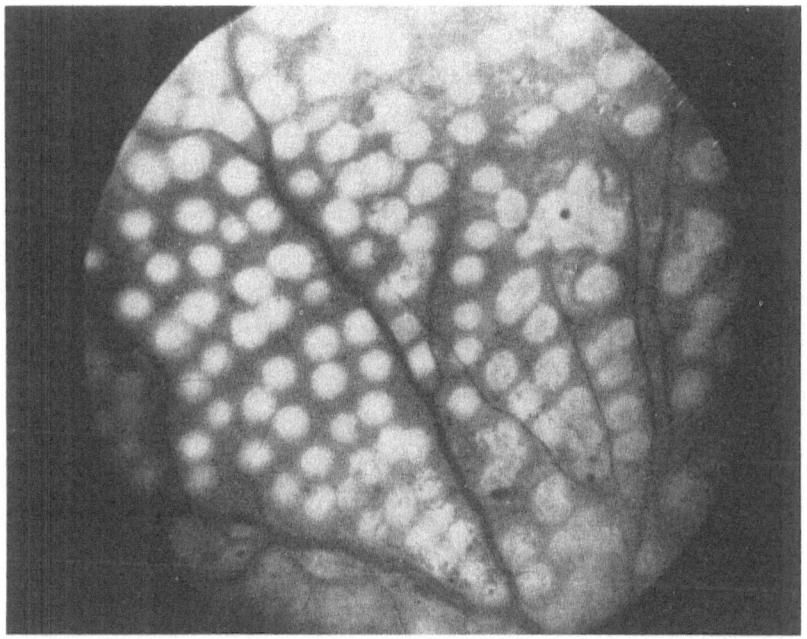

Fig. 6. Multiple peripheral ablative photocoagulation of eye depicated in Fig. 4 and 5.

effort should be made to encourage internists to refer all diabetic patients for ophthalmological evaluation and follow-up. Photocoagulation is indicated once proliferative retinopathy or macular involvement in nonproliferative retinopathy is detected.

Follow-up evaluation of the patient after treatment with argon laser photocoagulation for diabetic retinopathy is equally important. Since recurrent neovascularization is a common sequela, all patients treated for proliferative retinopathy should be re-evaluated with dilated fundus examination and with fluorescein angioscopy every two to three months during the first year following treatment and thereafter every four months.

SUMMARY

Argon laser slit lamp photocoagulation has been discussed as it applies to the management of diabetic retinopathy. The importance of feeder vessel treatment techniques using enlargements of arterial-phase-fluorescein angiograms is stressed. The use of multiple peripheral retinal photocoagulation is recommended to reduce the incidence of recurrent neovascularization. Continual evaluation of diabetic retinopathy both pre- and post-treatment is mandatory.

REFERENCES

AIELLO, L. M., BEETHAM, W. D., et al.: Ruby laser photocoagulation in treatment of diabetic proliferative retinopathy: preliminary report. In GOLDBERG, M. F. & FINE, S. L. (eds.) Symposium on Treatment of Diabetic Retinopathy. Arlington, Va., U.S. Dept. Health, Education and Welfare, pp. 437–463 (1968).

GOLDBERG, M. F. & FINE, S. L.: Symposium on Treatment of Diabetic Retinopathy. Arlington, Va., U.S. Dept. Health. Education and Welfare, Foreword (1968).

LITTLE, H. L., ZWENG, H. C. & PEABODY, R. R.: Argon laser slitlamp retinal photocoagulation. *Trans. Amer. Acad. Ophthal. Otolaryng.* 74: *85–97* (1970).

LITTLE, H. L. & ZWENG, H. C.: Complications of argon laser retinal photocoagulation. *Trans. Pac. Coast Oto-Ophthal. Soc.* 52: *115–129* (1971).

WESSING, A. K. & MEYER-SCHWICKERATH, G.: Results of photocoagulation in diabetic retinopathy. In Goldberg, M. F. and Fine, S. L., (eds.) Symposium on Treatment of Diabetic Retinopathy. Arlington, Va., U.S. Dept. Health, Education and Welfare, pp. 569–592 (1968).

WHITTINGTON, T. H.: Vitreous opacity and blindness in young diabetics. *Trans. Ophthal. Soc. U.K.* 84: *469–483* (1964).

ZWENG, H. C., LITTLE, H. L. & PEABODY, R. R.: Further observations in argon laser photocoagulation of diabetic retinopathy. *Trans. Amer. Acad. Ophthal. Otolaryng.* 76: *990–1003* (1972).

DIABETIC RETINOPATHY TREATMENT WITH ARGON-COAGULATION AND XENON-COAGULATION

G. MEYER-SCHWICKERATH

(*Essen*)

Out of several hundred patients treated with argon-coagulation 70% are cases with diabetic retinopathy. This shows that from our point of view diabetic retinopathy seems to be one of the major indications of argon-photocoagulation. On the other hand we have to mention that we have several thousand cases treated with xenon-coagulation alone or in combination with argon.

Our main indication is the treatment of isolated aneurysms close to the disk and close to the macula. They can be destroyed with very small fields of argon-coagulations without causing too much damage to the surrounding tissue. As a rule xenon-coagulation succeeds in edematous retina only down to a size of 3 or 1,5°, whereas argon-coagulation can succeed in much smaller coagulation fields.

In the periphery of normal cases of back-ground type of diabetic retinopathy we have found that xenon-coagulation is easier to perform and quicker than argon-coagulation. As stated before we feel that the production of larger fields is more difficult with argon than with xenon. In the periphery it is not desirable to take very small coagulations. The size of 1,5 or 3° is sufficient. This is the reason why we have performed in quite a number of cases xenon-coagulations in the periphery and subsequent argon-coagulations around the disc and the macular area.

This is important for cases in which the disappearance of diabetic changes in the centre does not occur after peripheral coagulation. In many cases however the coagulation of the centre itself is not necessary because the centre clears up when coagulations in the periphery have been performed. In those cases however where a tendency to proliferation, edema and yellowish deposits remains unchanged after peripheral coagulations, the isolated treatment of small aneurysms in the retinal centre has to be performed. This can be done more accurately with argon- than with xenon-coagulation.

One of the most interesting and important problems is the treatment of proliferating blood vessels. As stated in several reports we have recorded that after performance of peripheral photocoagulation it is extremely rare that the proliferative stage of diabetic retinopathy does occur at all. If however there is already a proliferation, we feel that peripheral argon- or xenon-coagulation should be performed in addition to direct treatment of proliferations, either from the disc or from the retinal periphery. In many pictures we have seen and recorded, that proliferations from the disc may disappear after peripheral photocoagulation has been performed.

In numerous cases we have tried to perform photocoagulation in nacked isolated vessels which run through the vitreous. We have never succeeded in occluding these vessels permanently. On the other hand, if there are several vessels close to each other we are able to get a contraction and, in some cases, to get an occlusion of proliferating blood vessels. If no peripheral coagulation has been performed, however, we have seen in almost all cases that the coagulated proliferation re-occurs after some weeks or months. For this reason we recommend that peripheral photocoagulation should be performed in almost all of these cases.

If the proliferation is still in the level or just above the level of the retina, normal photocoagulation either by xenon or by argon may succeed in destroying these proliferations.

I would like to draw your attention to the work of AMALRIC and WESSING, who have shown that peripheral diathermy should be performed in cases in which photocoagulation is not possible because of intraocular hemorrhage. In quite a number of these cases photocoagulation becomes possible later on and remarkable results may be obtained.

There is no doubt that photocoagulation is at present the most powerful weapon against diabetic retinopathy. It should however not attack the proliferating blood vessels alone. The best results are obtained either in the pure backgroundcases or in those in which proliferation is still in the level of the retina.

PREVENTING COMPLICATIONS IN ARGON
LASER RETINAL PHOTOCOAGULATION

HUNTER L. LITTLE, M.D.

(Palo Alto)

Complications have occurred from argon laser photocoagulation. LITTLE & ZWENG have documented incidents of corneal burn, lenticular burn, hemorrhage, preretinal membrane contracture, nerve fiber field defect, ischemic papillitis, and recurrent neovascularization (LITTLE & ZWENG). This paper provides a discussion of these complications and of methods to avoid them.

Five cases of corneal burns were experienced. Four consisted of minor superficial epithelial edema which cleared within 24 to 48 hours. One case resulted in ulceration of the anterior corneal stroma (Fig. 1). All occurred with the fifty and one-hundred micron spot sizes with power levels greater than five hundred milliwatts. In the severe burn, the power level was one watt. Exposure times were one to four seconds.

Elimination of corneal burns has been achieved by changes in the laser and in the optical train that conducts the beam into the eye. The beam diameter at the cornea was altered from 100 microns to 1000 microns while maintaining a 50 micron spot at the retina. The increased corneal beam diameter reduces the energy density of the laser beam at the cornea (Fig. 2).

One case of lenticular burn has been documented. It occurred in the same case with the severe corneal burn. The incident resulted with settings of 100 micron spot, 1000 milliwatts, and 1 second. The lenticular burns were discreet opacities in the anterior cortex (Fig. 1). They were observed at the time of coagulation, and no change in the opacity has occurred in a two year follow-up.

Since the manufacturer has made modifications of the instrument, corneal and lenticular burns have not been produced. Nevertheless, powers greater than 400 milliwatts should not be used with spot sizes less than 200 microns in diameter. The 100 micron spot still has the smallest beam diameter at the cornea; thus, it is the most hazardous setting with power levels over 400 milliwatts.

RETINAL HEMORRHAGE

Hemorrhage is the most frequent and disabling complication of argon laser retinal photocoagulation. Hemorrhage can be localized to the area of treatment,

Palo Alto Medical Clinic, Palo Alto Medical Research Foundation and Stanford University School of Medicine, Palo Alto, California.

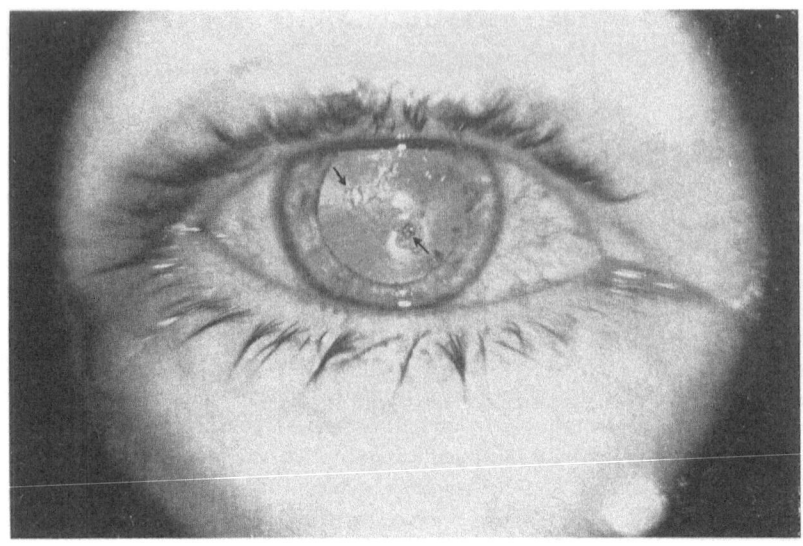

Fig. 1. Corneal and lenticular burns produced by high energy density argon laser beam. (50 to 100 micron spot size, 1000 milliwatts power, 4 seconds exposure time).

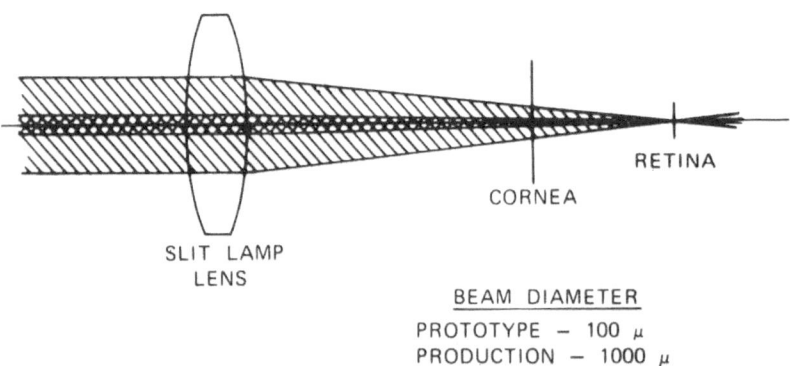

SLIT LAMP
LENS

BEAM DIAMETER
PROTOTYPE – 100 μ
PRODUCTION – 1000 μ

Fig. 2. Diagram illustrates argon laser beam diameter at cornea of 100 microns before alteration of instrument and of 1000 microns after alteration.

or it can be massive enough to obscure all fundus details. Bleeding from the time of treatment to one week after treatment is arbitrarily designated as a complication. Forty-six hemorrhages have occurred from treatment of 189 eyes with diabetic retinopathy; an average of three photocoagulation sessions were necessary for each eye. This represents a 24% incidence of hemorrhage per patient, or an 8% incidence of hemorrhage per treatment. Only 9 of the 46 hemorrhages were significant resulting in loss of vision, preretinal contrac-

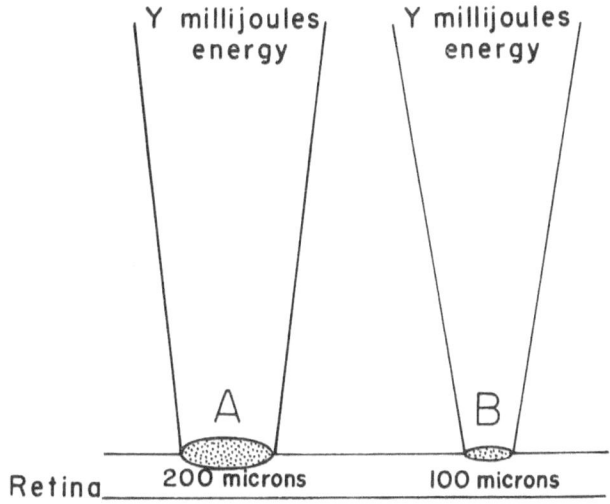

Area spot A = 4X spot B
∴ Energy density spot B = 4X spot A

Fig. 3. Theoretical comparison of energy density in relation to radius of spot size.
Energy density of spot B equals 4X spot A.

ture, recurrent growth of vessels, or retinal detachment. This represents an incidence for significant hemorrhage of 4.8% per eye and of 1.6% per treatment of proliferative retinopathy.

The understanding of power density is important in preventing hemorrhage. Power density is power per unit area. It varies inversely with the size of the photocoagulation beam on the retina. Thus, by reducing the beam diameter from 200 microns to 100 microns, the operator reduces the area 4 times. (Area equals πr^2.) If the power is unchanged, the power density is 4 times greater with the 100 micron beam diameter (Fig. 3).

In a biological medium with blood supply, the heat generated in the irradiated area is dispersed by surrounding tissue. A small spot is cooled more rapidly than a large spot since the center of the large spot is further from the cooling source. In practice, when the beam diameter is halved, the outpower of the laser must be halved.

Because of the high absorption properties of the argon laser beam by blood, such vascular occlusions produce immediate changes in the hemodynamics of retinal circulation. Sudden closure of venous or efferent channels causes vascular engorgement and hemorrhage. Thus, differentiation of arterial or afferent vessels from venous or efferent vessels is essential in reducing the complication of hemorrhage.

In proliferative retinopathies, the afferent and efferent vessels are difficult to differentiate because the usual color difference between arteries and veins may be absent, the vessels are intertwined among themselves, and the surrounding connective tissue obscures the view. Fluorescein angiography provides a method by which one can identify frequently the afferent vessels to neovascular fronds. Identification of feeder vessels is facilitated by enlarging the photographs, projecting the negatives, and obtaining stereo-angiograms.

By treating the feeder vessels, obliteration of neovascular fronds is accomplished with minimal risk of hemorrhage. With the 50 micron spot setting, precise microvascular surgery is achieved (Fig. 4, 5, 6). The large efferent vascular channels are avoided until the entire frond is totally obliterated. Repeated coagulation frequently is necessary within 24 hours to assure permanent closure of the frond.

Incidence of hemorrhage is reduced by sedentary activity during the 4 weeks post-treatment. Head elevation, stool softeners, sedatives when indicated, and abstinence from physical activity are recommended during this period. Occasionally pin hole glasses are used.

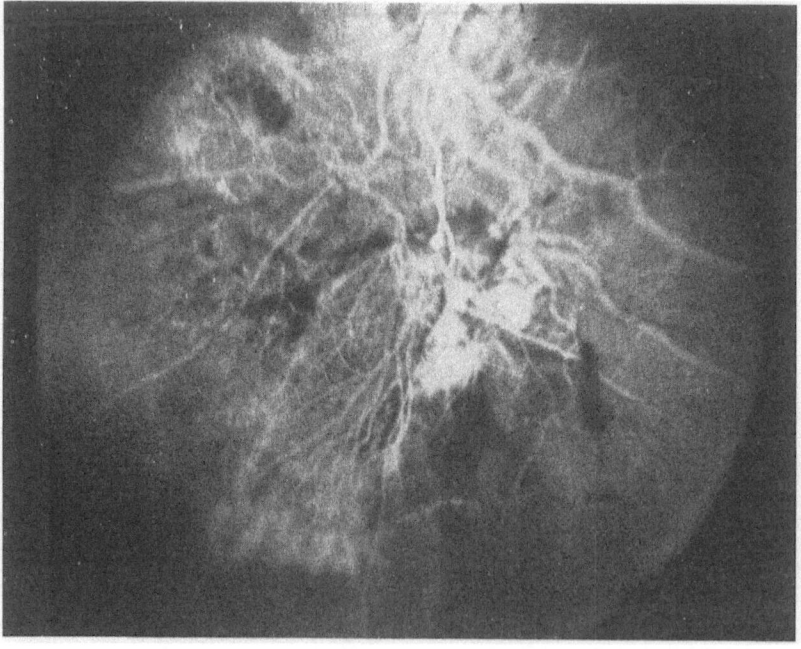

Fig. 4. Pretreatment fluorescein angiogram in venous phase shows large proliferative neovascular frond in diabetic.

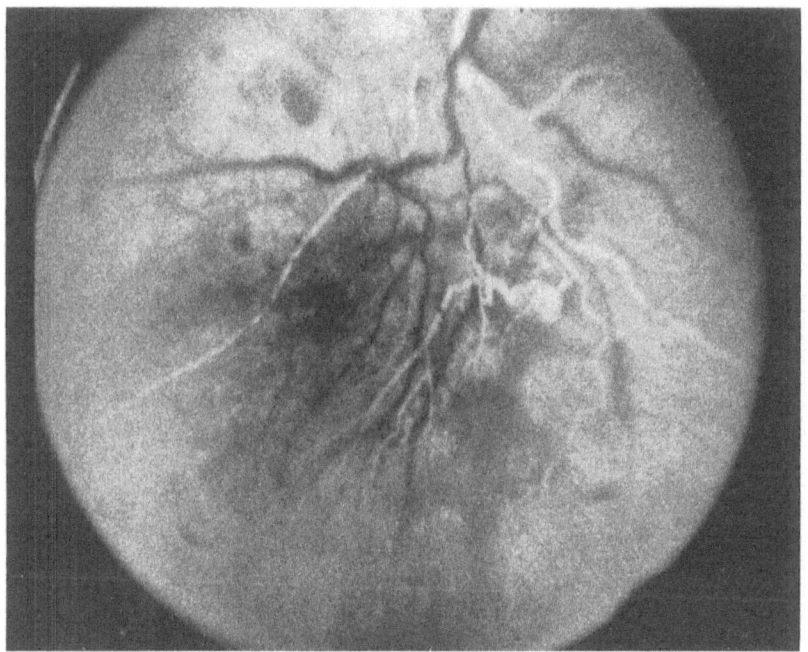

Fig. 5. Pretreatment arterial phase angiogram of case depicted in Fig. 4, shows arterial feed (white) and large efferent vessels (black).

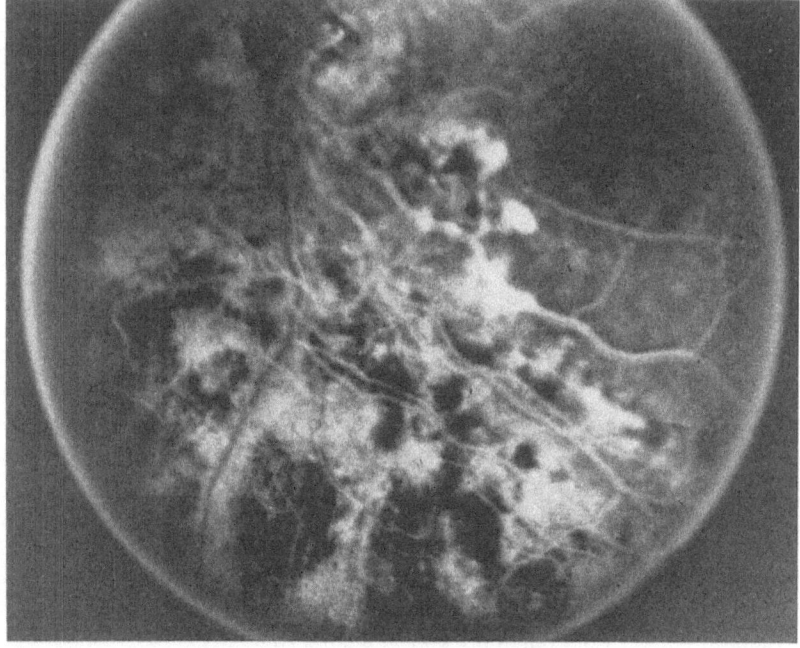

Fig. 6. One year post-treatment angiogram in venous phase shows obliteration of large frond depicted in Fig. 4.

Choroidal neovascularization is the primary cause of choroidal hemorrhages and hemorrhagic detachments of the retinal pigment epithelium. It occurs in senile choroidal macular degeneration and in histoplasmic choroiditis. Photocoagulation of choroidal neovascularization can prevent hemorrhage. However, if the photocoagulation intensity is minimal or if the area is incompletely treated, hemorrhage can result. High magnification of the choroidal and arterial phase angiograms delineate the area of choroidal neovascularization. Moderately heavy photocoagulation of the entire area of choroidal neovascularization usually eliminates the vascular leaks.

Complications in argon laser treatment of senile choroidal macular degeneration and histoplasmic choroiditis can be minimized by proper selection of cases to be treated. Favorable results occur in those cases with localized choroidal vascular leaks not involving the fovea, absence of cystoid degeneration of the sensory retina, and absence of disciform fibrous scar.

PRERETINAL MEMBRANE CONTRACTURE

Since preretinal membrane contracture occurs with some of the disease entities treated with argon laser, an accurate examination of the macula before treatment is essential. This is particularly true in diabetic retinopathy in which macular edema and preretinal striations frequently are present.

Preretinal membrane contracture has developed in 6 of 914 eyes treated between May 1969 and May 1972. All ensued treatment of macular lesions or retinal neovascularization in the posterior fundus. It has been observed following treatment of preretinal hemorrhage; the blood increases the absorption of the beam, thus heating of the internal limiting membrane and adjacent vitreous takes place.

The macular pucker syndrome has not been observed in the argon laser treatment of peripheral retinal pathology. This record does not preclude the possibility of this dreaded complication.

NERVE FIBER FIELD DEFECTS

Nerve fiber field defects have occurred in 8 cases (Fig. 7). These have usually followed repeated photocoagulation about the optic disc. In the 2 to 4 weeks following coagulation the retina becomes thin with the nerve fiber layer in closer proximity to the hyperplastic underlying retinal pigment epithelium. Hence, there is greater absorption of the light and greater heating of the nerve fiber bundles. Therefore, it is best to treat over the disc and not around its margin to treat preferably when the retina is of normal thickness rather than waiting until it becomes thin following previous coagulation (Fig. 8). This complication occurred only once with the initial treatment.

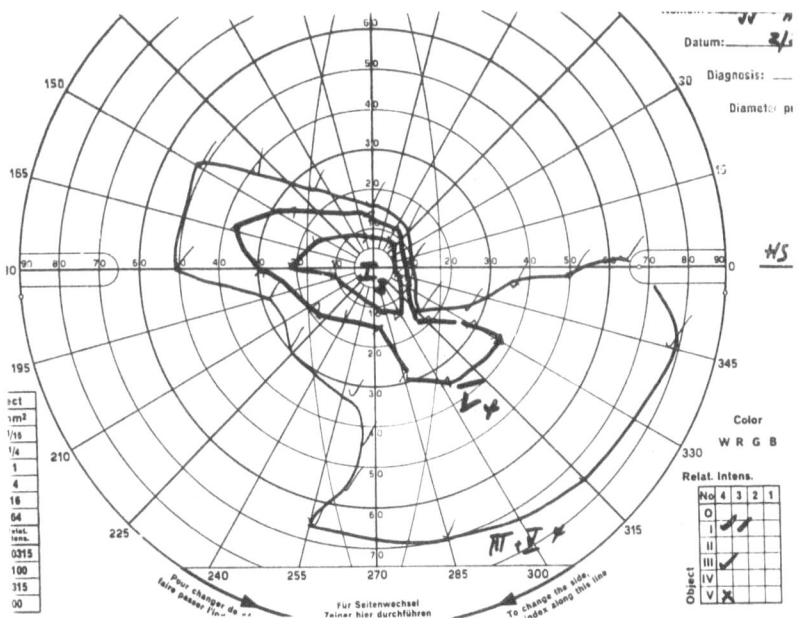

Fig. 7. Nerve fiber field defect following repeated laser photocoagulation about optic disc.

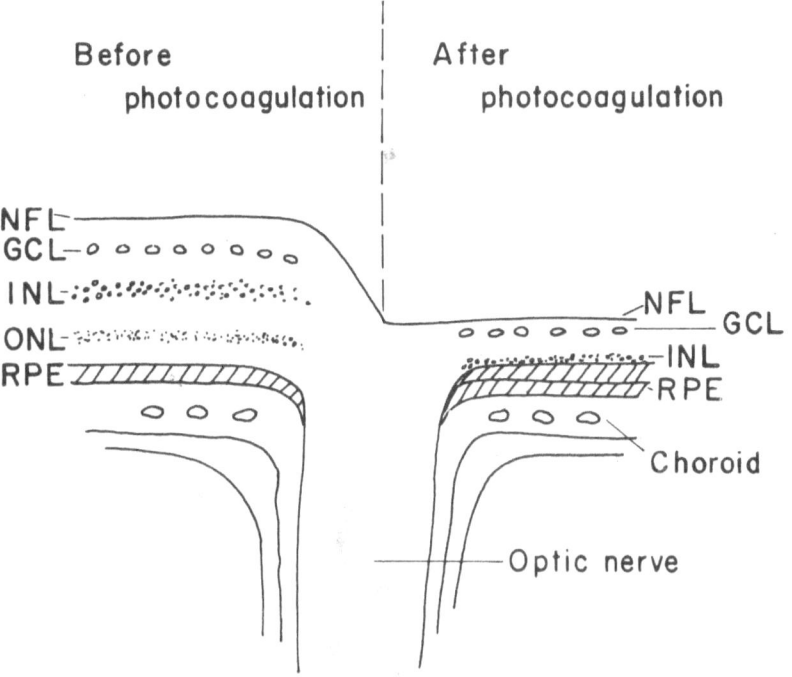

Fig. 8. Diagram illustrates close proximity of nerve fiber layer to hyperplastic retinal pigment epithelium in scarred retina after previous photocoagulation.

Two cases of ischemic papillitis have occurred with very heavy argon laser photocoagulation directed over the nervehead itself. Both were observed within 24 hours following coagulation over the nervehead with 500 milliwatts of power, one to 2 seconds exposure times and 100 to 200 micron spot sizes. Both had Marcus Gunn pupillary phenomena and pale swollen nerveheads. Both showed dramatic recovery of visual acuity within one week following onset of the papillitis. Steroids were given. When treating on the disc, the beam should be focused on the abnormal vessels. With beams larger than 100 microns, unnecessary heating of the optic disc is likely to result. If power levels are kept below 200 milliwatts spot size below 100 microns, and exposure times not more than .2 sec. ischemic papillitis should not occur.

RECURRENT RETINAL NEOVASCULARIZATION

Two to 6 months after treatment recurrent neovascular tufts have developed adjacent to previously treated areas (Fig. 9). In 36% of proliferative diabetic retinopathies with treatment to the frond only, recurrent neovascularization ensues. The occurrence alerts the ophthalmologist of the need for continued

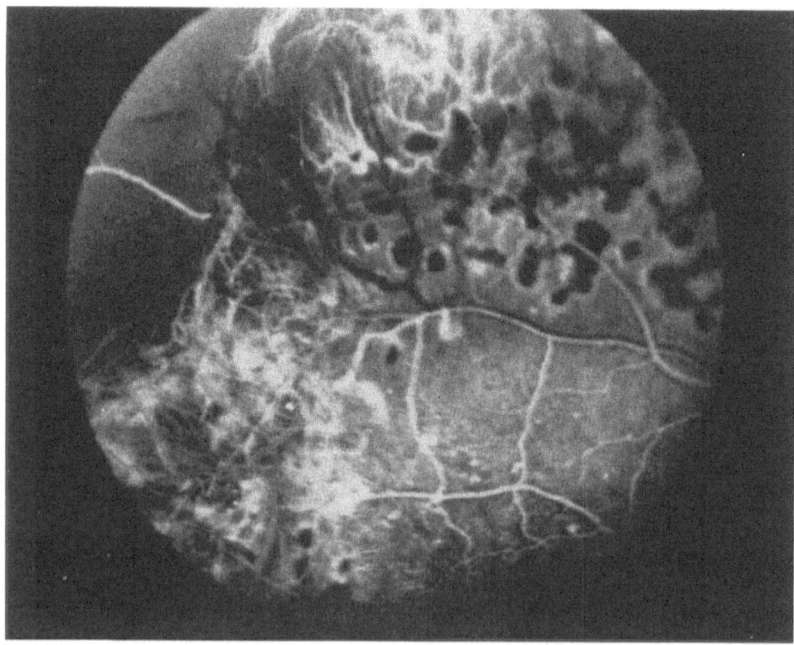

Fig. 9. Angiogram shows recurrent neovascularization in diabetic patient peripheral to area treated 3 months previously.

observation of patients with diseases prone to retinal neovascularization. The stimulus for recurrent proliferation of vessels can be minimized by surrounding the area under treatment with a ring of coagulation in an attempt to produce retinal necrosis, thus avoiding relative hypoxia and stimulation of neovascularization. Retinal ablation with 1000 to 1500 lesions provides the best method to minimize recurrent retinal neovascularization.

SUMMARY

Complications encountered in the treatment of 914 eyes with the argon laser photocoagulator are discussed. Methods by which these complications can be prevented or minimized are discussed.

REFERENCES

LITTLE, H. L. & ZWENG, H. C.: Complications of argon laser retinal photocoagulation. *Trans. Pac. Coast Oto-Ophthal. Soc.* 52: *115–129*.

Key Words:
Complications
Argon laser retinal photocoagulation
Corneal burn
Lenticular burn
Hemorrhage
Afferent (feeder) vessels
Efferent vessels
Fluorescein angiography
Preretinal membrane contracture
Nerve fiber field defect
Ischemic papillitis
Recurrent neovascularization
Retinal ablation